FOOD AND BEVERAGE CONSUMPTION AND HEALTH

CAFFEINE

CONSUMPTION, SIDE EFFECTS AND IMPACT ON PERFORMANCE AND MOOD

FOOD AND BEVERAGE CONSUMPTION AND HEALTH

Additional books in this series can be found on Nova's website under the Series tab.

Additional e-books in this series can be found on Nova's website under the e-book tab.

FOOD AND BEVERAGE CONSUMPTION AND HEALTH

CAFFEINE

CONSUMPTION, SIDE EFFECTS AND IMPACT ON PERFORMANCE AND MOOD

AIMÉE S. TOLLEY
EDITOR

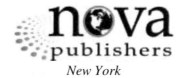

New York

Copyright © 2014 by Nova Science Publishers, Inc.

All rights reserved. No part of this book may be reproduced, stored in a retrieval system or transmitted in any form or by any means: electronic, electrostatic, magnetic, tape, mechanical photocopying, recording or otherwise without the written permission of the Publisher.

For permission to use material from this book please contact us:
Telephone 631-231-7269; Fax 631-231-8175
Web Site: http://www.novapublishers.com

NOTICE TO THE READER

The Publisher has taken reasonable care in the preparation of this book, but makes no expressed or implied warranty of any kind and assumes no responsibility for any errors or omissions. No liability is assumed for incidental or consequential damages in connection with or arising out of information contained in this book. The Publisher shall not be liable for any special, consequential, or exemplary damages resulting, in whole or in part, from the readers' use of, or reliance upon, this material. Any parts of this book based on government reports are so indicated and copyright is claimed for those parts to the extent applicable to compilations of such works.

Independent verification should be sought for any data, advice or recommendations contained in this book. In addition, no responsibility is assumed by the publisher for any injury and/or damage to persons or property arising from any methods, products, instructions, ideas or otherwise contained in this publication.

This publication is designed to provide accurate and authoritative information with regard to the subject matter covered herein. It is sold with the clear understanding that the Publisher is not engaged in rendering legal or any other professional services. If legal or any other expert assistance is required, the services of a competent person should be sought. FROM A DECLARATION OF PARTICIPANTS JOINTLY ADOPTED BY A COMMITTEE OF THE AMERICAN BAR ASSOCIATION AND A COMMITTEE OF PUBLISHERS.

Additional color graphics may be available in the e-book version of this book.

Library of Congress Cataloging-in-Publication Data

ISBN: 978-1-63117-777-4

Published by Nova Science Publishers, Inc. † New York

CONTENTS

Preface		**vii**
Chapter 1	Too Late for Tea Time? The Potential of Use of Caffeine for Health in the Elderly *E. Paul Cherniack*	**1**
Chapter 2	Caffeine Facilitates Conditioned Operant Responses Associated with Self-Administration of High Fat Foods in Rats *Xiu Liu*	**19**
Chapter 3	Caffeine: Forms of Consumption, Toxicity, Therapeutic Effects and Their Use in Medicine *A. Martín, E. Montial, M. Iturbe, A. Quintano, B. Fernández-Miret, M. Prieto, H. Barrasa, S. Castaño, E. Jiménez, F. J. Maynar, N. Ruiz, E. Corral, G. Balziskueta, S. Cabañes and F. Fonseca*	**35**
Chapter 4	Caffeine Modulation of Alcohol Intake: Impact on Its Psychomotor Effects and Withdrawal. *M. Correa, N. San Miguel, L. López-Cruz, P. Bayarri and J. D. Salamone*	**89**
Chapter 5	Regulation Mechanism of Caffeine on Glucose Transport and Upstream Signaling Pathways in Skeletal Muscle *Tatsuro Egawa, Satoshi Tsuda, Taku Hamada, Katsumasa Goto and Tatsuya Hayashi*	**113**

Chapter 6	Utilization Efficiency Improvement of Tea Leaves' Biological Potential as a Result of SC-CO_2 Pretreatment	139
	F. M. Gumerov, Truong Nam Hung, F. N. Shamsetdinov, Z. I. Zaripov, F. R. Gabitov and B. Le Neindre	
Index		**203**

PREFACE

Caffeine is a natural substance that is present in over 60 plant species. Alternative names include theine, guaranine and mateine. It is consumed by humans in the form of beverages such as coffee, tea, chocolate and soft drinks. Coffee was first discovered in Arabia during the 9th century, and was originally cultivated in Ethiopia. Tea was first drunk in China and cacao was discovered in South America. During the 15th century, coffee became popular all over the world. The most common species of coffee are Coffea arabica (Arabica coffee) and Coffea canephora (Robusta coffee), which respectively account for 80-90% and 10-20% of worldwide production. Coffee is the product which contains the highest and most variable quantity of caffeine in the human diet. This book discusses more about the consumption of caffeine, the side effects it may have on the human body, and its impact of an individual's performance and mood once consumed.

Chapter 1 – Caffeine has long been studied for its effects on physical performance, but few studies have been conducted specifically in elderly individuals. In several short-term trials, older individuals who used caffeine improved in some but not all measures of exercise performance, but the results may have been confounded by the influences of habitual caffeine use and withdrawal. The mechanism by which caffeine might influence improvement in exercise is not entirely known, nor is it certain whether caffeine acts on the muscle or affects perception of exercise-related pain and fatigue. Caffeine might also theoretically retard the development of cognitive impairment in the elderly and depression. Epidemiologic studies suggest an association between caffeine consumption and incidence or progression of dementia and depression, which may be stronger for women than men. No prospective trials of have been published using caffeine to treat cognition, and one small trial outlined an effect on mood in older persons. Future studies should clarify the effects, synergies and confounders, and elucidate the optimum form and timing of administration.

Chapter 2 – In light of the fact that the authors' previous research showed that caffeine facilitated the behavioral motivation effect of an environmental cue conditioned to nicotine self-administration (Liu and Jernigan 2012), the present study was designed to examine the issue of whether the enhancing effect of caffeine on conditioned reinforcement extends to behavior supported by a cue previously conditioned to a natural reward food. Male Sprague-Dawley rats, satiated with standard laboratory chow, were trained to self-administer food pellets containing high fat contents on a progressive ratio schedule of reinforcement. Each pellet delivery was associated with a sensory stimulus so that the later acquired incentive value and become a food-conditioned cue. After lever responses were extinguished by withholding food pellet and its cue, effects of caffeine (5 mg/kg, i.p.) administration alone or together with re-presentation of food cue on lever responses were examined in the test sessions where responses did not result in delivery of food pellets. Re-presentations of the food cue effectively reinstated extinguished responses on the previously active, food-reinforced lever. Although pre-session administration of caffeine on its own did not increase responses, caffeine significantly potentiated the cue-induced reinstatement of food-seeking responses. These data demonstrate that acute caffeine administration can facilitate the behavioral motivation effect of natural reward (food) conditioned stimuli. This finding suggests that caffeine consumption may heighten food-seeking behavior triggered by exposure to the food-associated environmental stimuli.

Chapter 3 – Caffeinated drinks (coffee and others) and tea are the most consumed, socially-acceptable stimulants in the world. In their natural forms, coffee and tea contain several chemical components that may confer both beneficial and adverse health effects,

Caffeine, a methylxanthine, is closely related to theophylline. Caffeine is rapidly and completely absorbed from the gastrointestinal tract. The volume of distribution in adults is approximately 0.5 L/kg. Caffeine is primarily metabolized by the cytochrome P450 (CYP) oxidase system in the liver. The plasma half-life of caffeine varies considerably from person to person, with an average half-life of 5-8 hours in healthy, nonsmoking adults. Caffeine clearance is accelerated in smokers; clearance is slowed in pregnancy, in liver disease, and in the presence of some CYP inhibitors.

There is insufficient evidence for promoting or discouraging coffee consumption in the daily diet. Caffeine consumption has multiple systemic effects, involving the neuropsychiatric, cardiovascular, endocrine-metabolic, genitourinary and gastrointestinal systems. The impact on health may be modified by genetic factors, age, sex, medications, and other environmental exposures.

It is used for treating of idiopathic apnea of prematurity, acute respiratory depression, restore mental alertness o wakefulness when experiencing fatigue, and less frequently for treating spinal puncture headache, diuretic, augmentation of seizure induction during electroconvulsive therapy, and acute migraine (combined with indomethacyn and prochlorperazine).

This review will focus on the consumption of caffeine, its role on neurologic performance, sport and some specific disease processes, explaining side effects, toxicity, caffeine dependence, withdrawal and tolerance.

Chapter 4 – The impact of caffeine on ethanol consumption and abuse has become a topic of great interest due to the rise in popularity of "energy drinks". Energy drinks have many different components, although the main active ingredient is caffeine. These drinks are frequently taken in combination with alcohol under the belief that caffeine can offset some of the intoxicating effects of ethanol. However, scientific research has not universally supported the idea that caffeine can reduce the effects of ethanol in humans or in rodents, and the mechanisms mediating caffeine-ethanol interactions are not well understood. Caffeine and ethanol have a common biological substrate; both act on neurochemical processes related to the neuromodulator adenosine. Caffeine acts as a non-selective adenosine A_1 and A_{2A} receptor antagonist, while ethanol has been demonstrated to increase the basal adenosinergic tone via multiple mechanisms. Since adenosine transmission modulates multiple behavioral processes, the interaction of both drugs can regulate a wide range of behavioral effects, which can have an impact on alcohol consumption and the development of alcohol addiction. In the present review the authors discuss epidemiological studies and laboratory animal work that have assessed the impact of caffeine on alcohol consumption. In addition, they evaluate how caffeine can also affect the consumption of other drugs of abuse. Finally the authors present data on human and animal studies analyzing the impact of caffeine on alcohol withdrawal, and psychomotor performance.

Chapter 5 – Skeletal muscle is the major organ playing an important role in whole-body glucose metabolism. Caffeine (1,3,7-trimethylxanthine) has been implicated in the regulation of skeletal muscle glucose metabolism, including insulin-dependent and -independent glucose transport. However, the precise mechanism of how caffeine modulates these phenomena has not been firmly established. In this review, the authors provide their recent experimental evidence linking caffeine to glucose transport and upstream signaling pathways in skeletal muscle.

The initial part of this chapter introduced the effect of caffeine on insulin-dependent signaling pathways of glucose transport in skeletal muscle.

Incubation of isolated muscle with caffeine suppressed insulin-dependent tyrosine phosphorylation of insulin receptor substrate (IRS)-1. This response was accompanied with inhibition of insulin-dependent signaling pathways; phosphorylation of phosphatidylinositol-3 kinase and Akt, and with inhibition of insulin-dependent glucose transport. In addition, caffeine enhanced phosphorylation of IRS-1 on the inhibitory site Ser[307] and inhibitor-κB kinase (IKK). Suppression of the IKK/IRS-1 Ser[307] cascade reduced the caffeine-mediated downregulation of IRS-1 tyrosine phosphorylation and insulin-dependent glucose transport. On the other hand, Ca^{2+} release inhibitor, dantrolene did not rescue the downregulations while suppressing 5'AMP-activated protein kinase (AMPK)/IRS-1 Ser[789] cascade.

Intravenous injection of caffeine at a physiological dose (5 mg/kg) in rats inhibited the insulin-dependent IRS-1 tyrosine phosphorylation and Akt phosphorylation in skeletal muscle. The findings indicate that caffeine inhibits insulin-dependent glucose transport through IRS-1 dysfunction, IKK/IRS-1 Ser[307]-dependently and Ca^{2+}- and AMPK-independently, in skeletal muscle.

The second part of this chapter introduced how caffeine acts on AMPK and which α isoform of AMPK (AMPKα1 and AMPKα2) is predominantly activated by caffeine in skeletal muscle. Incubation of rat skeletal muscles with caffeine at high doses (3 mM) resulted in cellular energy deprivation and activation of both AMPKα1 and AMPKα2, and Ca^{2+}/calmodulin-dependent protein kinase (CaMK) II. Caffeine stimulation at low dose (1 mM) did not cause energy deprivation and activation of AMPKα2 or CaMKII, but did activate AMPKα1. Intravenous injection of caffeine (5 mg/kg) in rat preferentially activated AMPKα1 in epitrochlearis muscle.

The findings indicate that caffeine activates AMPK and CaMKII in skeletal muscle through either an energy-dependent or -independent pathway, and AMPKα1 plays a pivotal role in insulin-independent glucose transport in physiological conditions.

The findings of these investigations provide valuable information about the regulation mechanism underlying the caffeine-induced metabolic changes that occur in skeletal muscle.

Chapter 6 – The pretreatment of commercial samples of Vietnamese and Chinese green teas shows that it is possible to increase the extractability of chemical, including caffeine, in aqueous phase at the stage of beverage concoction and provide more complete information of biological potential of the feedstock. Procedures are proposed for an extract of raw materials in ($SC\text{-}CO_2$) medium; ($SC\text{-}CO_2$) circulation through the processed raw materials, multiple decompressions in ($SC\text{-}CO_2$) medium, containing processed raw materials. For example, the circulation of carbon dioxide during 4 hours through the extractor with the feedstock at $T = 333.15K$ and $P = 10$ MPa provides 25% increased caffeine yield, into the aqueous phase, at the stage of beverage concoction. The conditions to minimize the effect of ($SC\text{-}CO_2$) extraction, upon minerals and biologically active components of tea leaves are investigated in the implementation of these procedures In particular, the study of solubility of caffeine in supercritical carbon dioxide in the temperature range $T = 308.15\text{-}333.15$ K and the pressure range $P = 7\text{-}30$ MPa, shows that the pressure range of 7-11 MPa gives optimal results for ($SC\text{-}CO_2$) flowing through the processing raw materials. The results of research of the other factors, related to the procedure, and properties of the corresponding thermodynamic systems are presented; there are required for the mathematical modeling of the operating process, in order to serve as a basis for designing the future large scale equipment. In particular, the behavior of the following properties has been investigated: the enthalpy of mixing for (caffeine - $SC\text{-}CO_2$) systems and (cellulose - $SC\text{-}CO_2$) systems at 308.15K, 323.15K, 348.15K isotherms in the pressure range 0-40 MPa and 8-22 MPa, respectively. The isobaric heat capacity and density of (caffeine - carbon dioxide) mixtures; as well as some properties of the ternary system, containing (caffeine, carbon dioxide and water) are carried out. The results of the influence of the pretreatment on the composition and structure of tea leaves, cellulose and caffeine are presented. The results of solubility data and some useful properties of thermodynamic systems are reported.

In: Caffeine
Editor: Aimée S. Tolley

ISBN: 978-1-63117-777-4
© 2014 Nova Science Publishers, Inc.

Chapter 1

TOO LATE FOR TEA TIME? THE POTENTIAL OF USE OF CAFFEINE FOR HEALTH IN THE ELDERLY

E. Paul Cherniack

The Geriatrics institute, Division of Geriatrics and Gerontology,
Miller School of Medicine, University of Miami
and the Bruce W. Carter Miami VA Medical Center, US

ABSTRACT

Caffeine has long been studied for its effects on physical performance, but few studies have been conducted specifically in elderly individuals. In several short-term trials, older individuals who used caffeine improved in some but not all measures of exercise performance, but the results may have been confounded by the influences of habitual caffeine use and withdrawal. The mechanism by which caffeine might influence improvement in exercise is not entirely known, nor is it certain whether caffeine acts on the muscle or affects perception of exercise-related pain and fatigue. Caffeine might also theoretically retard the development of cognitive impairment in the elderly and depression. Epidemiologic studies suggest an association between caffeine consumption and incidence or progression of dementia and depression, which may be stronger for women than men. No prospective trials of have been published using caffeine to treat cognition, and one small trial outlined an effect on mood in older persons. Future studies should clarify the effects, synergies and confounders, and elucidate the optimum form and timing of administration.

INTRODUCTION: CAFFEINE USE IN THE ELDERLY

The worldwide popularity of caffeinated beverages needs no introduction, however, surprisingly little is known about their use by the elderly. Almost two decades ago, a survey noted coffee and tea are the most commonly consumed beverages by the elderly. Caffeine consumption declines by 25% in those over 70 from those aged 50-69 to 190mg caffeine daily (approximately the dose in a strong cup of coffee. [1] Caffeine pharmacokinetics and metabolism do not appear to change with age. [1] Age does appear to have limited influence on caffeine's physiologic effects, including an accentuation of urine volume and calcium excretion, and an increase in blood pressure. [1]

CAFFEINE AND PHYSICAL PERFORMANCE IN THE ELDERLY

Caffeine has long been studied for its effects on physical performance. Ingestion of caffeine increases the ability of trained athletes and military personnel to perform numerous tasks involving rigorous physical activity. [2] In such individuals, including athletes such as cyclists, runners, weightlifters, and participants in team sports, limited duration ingestion of caffeine induces short-term gains in exercise-related tasks. These enhancements following caffeine use consist of improved ability to perform standardized athletic tests, endurance, sprinting, and specific sports-related tasks. [3] Many, but not all studies have confirmed an effect, which is more pronounced after short-term ingestion in athletes who do not habitually use caffeine. [4, 5].

Few studies have been conducted specifically in elderly individuals. The first trial, a double-blinded placebo controlled, crossover investigation, took place almost one decade ago in Denmark. [6] In this investigation, 30 subjects at least age 70 (mean age 74.7) who consumed a mean of four and half cups of coffee a day were first asked to withhold caffeine ingestion for two days. Next, they were given a dose of either 6mg/kg caffeine or a placebo. Sixty minutes later, participants engaged in a series of tests including standing on a dynamometer platform, cycling on a cycle ergometer, walking (to measure gait speed), and measurement of movement and reaction times. The balance measurements on the platform included standing balance with or without eyes closed, and semitandem stance. In reaction time assessments, subjects had to remove their hand from a button and depress a second button upon viewing a light.

Participants next ate a sandwich and a drink, after which they waited thirty minutes. Subjects then flexed their arms against a strain gage attached to a dynamometer. Following a fifteen minute break, subjects had to flex their arms to oppose a force of half maximal strength, with measurement of the length of time they maintained flexion. Participants performed the crossover experiment a week later.

Individuals who consumed caffeine significantly increased their endurance during cycle ergometry (p=.00001), augmented their isometric maximal strength (p<.00001), and reduced their perceived effort after five minutes (p=.02) and postural sway. Other parameters measured did not differ between subjects who consumed caffeine or a placebo.

While the study importantly documents a possible benefit to caffeine use in physical performance for elderly persons, the characteristics of the studied population suggests a confounding limitation to its applicability. Since heavy caffeine users were asked to abstain from drinking coffee for two days before being given a dose of caffeine, the study may have demonstrated the response of caffeine ingestion to caffeine withdrawal rather than imply the potential benefit of caffeine to naïve elderly individuals who exercise.

In another investigation, nineteen non-institutionalized older persons, at least age 65, performed a six-minute walk test after they consumed 200ml of coffee or tea with a mean caffeine dose of 29mg, a placebo drink, or exercise. [7] The time between consumption and exercise was not recorded. There was no difference in results of the test between individuals who took caffeine or those who did not, but the study was not designed to detect a difference between the two conditions.

In a third study, twelve older persons, ages 60 to 79, who habitually took an average of 100.2 mg/day of caffeine and abstained for two days, performed a test of cognitive perception (coincidence anticipation timing [CAT]), a test of mood (Brunel Mood State Inventory) and isokinetic knee extensions measured by a dynamometer. They subsequently consumed 3mg/kg caffeine or a placebo, waited one hour, and repeated the tests. [8] Subjects performed significantly better on the CAT test after caffeine (p=0.045) and on the "vigor" subscale of the Brunel inventory (p=.0009), but not on any of the other measured assessed. Again, as in the previous study, the two day period of abstention in habitual caffeine consumers may have confounded the results.

In one investigation, a much shorter period of abstinence was used. In this trial, thirty normal older persons, who were at least age 70, mean age 74.1, took a 6mg/kg dose of caffeine or a placebo. [9]

One hour later, they flexed their arms, their maximal isometric endurance and strength being measured by a dynamometer, and pedaled a cycle ergometer. Unfortunately, caffeine did improve any measure of physical function. The participants in this trial however, had a rather high mean coffee intake of six cups a day, which is not typical of the general older population, and the abstinence period of eight hours was short.

A significant and intriguing question that has yet to be resolved is the mechanism of caffeine's action on physical performance. The numerous hypotheses can be divided into two general categories: those that suggest that caffeine acts on muscle, and those that suggest that caffeine's effect is primarily cognitive, resulting in an altered perception of exercise. The possibility exists that caffeine may act through multiple mechanisms. Unfortunately, all of the potential mechanisms and whether age alters potential mechanisms of action all need further study.

Caffeine may enhance exercise by increasing aerobic work. In a recent investigation, seven participants, who were athletes, mean age 32.3, pedaled a stationary bicycle the equivalent of four kilometers following an initially exercise designed to lower participant's carbohydrate concentrations. [10] Subjects consuming caffeine averted decrement in cycling performance and aerobic work that occurred in a carbohydrate-deprived state.

Ingestion of caffeine may benefit exercise by lowering muscle interstitial potassium concentrations. [11] In one study, twelve athletes completed an exercise regimen which consisted of a series of four three minute sets of knee extensions following ingestion of 6mg/kg of caffeine or a placebo. Caffeine enabled subject to perform more work while intramuscular potassium concentrations were reduced, which they authors hypothesized lowered myocyte potassium efflux, resulting in less muscle fatigue.

Other mechanisms, such as alterations in the regulation of myocyte intracellular calcium or calcium channels, may explain caffeine's physiological effects, [12] such as greater maximal isokinetic muscle contractions, maximal muscle twitch, and voluntary muscular isometric contractions. [13] Within the myocyte, caffeine, by inhibiting phosphodiesterase, increases the production of cyclic AMP and GMP which, in turn regulates nitro oxide (NO) synthesis. NO facilitates myocyte calcium channel activity and induces the expression of genes which prevent apoptosis. [14] Nitric oxide synthetase enhances muscle contractile force, possibly by promoting glucose entry into muscle or calcium efflux from the sarcoplasmic reticulum. [14] In rat, caffeine injection changes NO isoform concentrations and the expression of the apoptotic regulatory gene Bcl12 in both skeletal muscle and myocardium. [14, 15] However, *in vivo*, the human serum caffeine concentrations that would be necessary to induce alterations of calcium flux may be so large that they could not feasible occur at doses that would not cause toxicity. [12] Another possibility, perhaps more likely, is that caffeine influences the perception of exercise.

Caffeine might, firstly, decrease the perception of pain during exercise. In one investigation, eleven athletes ingested 5mg/kg caffeine or a placebo and did one repetition of an exercise consisting of five minutes of cycle ergometry, lifting a weight, a bench press, and a back squat. [16] Participants rated their pain from 0 to 10 and their perceived exertion from 6 to 20. Caffeine consumption resulted in significantly less pain perception for all the exercises tested (p=0.02), while ingesting a placebo induced a significant reduction in pain perception for weight lifting only. In another trial, nine women had an electrical stimulation of leg muscles to elicit pain and muscle damage, and on the following day, a 5mg/kg dose of caffeine or placebo. [17] One hour later they exercised the damaged leg muscle by flexing it against resistance, and recorded pain perceived on a 0-100 pain intensity scale. Caffeine significantly reduced pain by a mean 12.7 units on the visual analogue scale (p=.036).

However, two other studies failed to confirm that caffeine modifies pain perception. In one, athletes drank 5mg/kg on 2 days of a caffeinated beverage or a placebo and cycled 10km on a cycle ergometer. [18] Caffeine did not change pain perception but did improve subjective perception on a pleasure/displeasure scale. Ten women who consumed 6m/kg caffeine did not report improved pain perception, but increased their performance at cycle ergometry. [19] Possibly, documentation of caffeine's modulation of pain perception may be contingent on the intensity, modality, and timing of the stimulus, and the instrument used to measure pain.

In addition, caffeine might reduce the perception of effort during exercise. In one trial, fifteen young volunteers ingested 6mg/kg caffeine or a placebo, after which they cycled for 30 minutes. [20] They rated exertion after the session on a 0-10 scale. Caffeine consumption resulted in a small but statistically significant decrement in perception of exertion (p<0.05).

CAFFEINE EFFECTS ON COGNITION IN THE ELDERLY

Caffeine's effect on the mind may extend beyond its role in exercise to other aspects of cognitive function such as alertness, mood, and memory. [21] Many animal studies have outlined the potential of caffeine to enhance cognition.

Numerous rodent studies have delineated the effect of caffeine on memory. Caffeine acts multiple neural pathways including several neurotransmitter systems, including the dopaminergic, cholinergic, and serotonergic systems. [22] In one investigation, rats were fed either two different concentrations of coffee, two different concentrations of caffeine, or a control diet. [23] Rats that consumed caffeine in any form performed better on object recognition and maze tests of memory and had increased levels of antioxidant enzymes.

Several studies have suggested a role for adenosine receptors in the effect of caffeine on the brain. In one investigation in which dementia was experimentally induced in rats, caffeine pretreatment alleviated the extent of dementia and augmented adenosine A_{2A} receptor density. [24] An additional study of the influence of caffeine on attention in rats demonstrated that caffeine's action on adenosine receptors mediated the effect. [25] Caffeine, through its activation of a kinase that prevents apoptosis, cyclic adenosine monophosphate-dependent kinase A, augments cyclic AMP levels and inhibits phosphodiesterase. In a mouse model of dementia, caffeine treatment prevented the formation of amyloid plaques and improved performance on maze memory tests. [26] Caffeine administration averted deficiency in olfactory discrimination in rats, which was mediated through A_1 and A_2 adenosine receptors. [27]

The application of caffeine *in vitro* averts neuronal death, and intraperitoneal administration or ingestion of caffeine prevents cognitive deficits induced by intracranial administration of amyloid fragments in mice. [28-31] Caffeine alleviated decrements in rodent maze test results induced by stress and high-fat high carbohydrate diets. [32]

The cognitive benefit of long-term caffeine consumption by young rats as evidenced by their performance on memory tests persisted into middle and old age. [33, 34] The benefits of both short- and long –term caffeine administration, including object recognition and avoidance memory in mice, has been associated with concentrations of tyrosine kinase receptor and brain-derived neurotrophic factor. [34, 35]

Caffeine might also enhance memory by improving mitochondrial function. [36] In one investigation, caffeine alleviated mitochondrial dysfunction in a transgenic mouse model of dementia. Caffeine may help mitochondria to reduce their production of reactive oxygen species (ROS). [36] Rabbits induced to develop brain amyloid plaques through ingestion of a high cholesterol diet that were fed caffeine had lower concentrations of ROS markers in their brains. [37]

Alternatively, or, perhaps in addition, the benefit of caffeine may be mediated by caffeine's action on the choroid plexus and enhancement of cerebrospinal fluid (CSF) production. In rats, chronic caffeine consumption increased CSF output by the choroid plexus with greater amyloid clearance. [38]

Caffeine may alleviate dementing illness by creating alterations of the blood-brain barrier. A number of studies attribute dysfunction of the blood-brain barrier in the pathogenesis of Alzheimer's disease, and caffeine, through inhibition of cell membrane receptors for adenosine and calcium transport, stabilize the blood-brain barrier. [39] Caffeine ingestion in a drug-induced rabbit and mouse dementia modes prevented seepage of a dye through the blood-brain barrier, and preserved concentration of tight junction proteins. [40, 41]

Alterations of sleep created by caffeine may have cognitive implications. Treatment of rats with caffeine averted deficits in cognition created by sleep deprivation and synapse connectivity. [42]

Finally, caffeine might impact cognition through epigenetic effects. [43] Caffeine has not been demonstrated yet to be an epigenetic modulator, but adenosine receptors may be involved in the epigenetic regulation and the pathogenesis of dementing illness. [43]

Human studies have also outlined the potential of caffeine to impact cognition in the elderly.

For many years, investigations have delineated short-term effects on human cognition. In one trial in younger individuals, ingestion of 200mg of caffeine improved attention measured by reaction time and alleviated fatigue on the Profile of Mood States questionnaire. [44] A dose of 240mg of caffeine administered to young adult volunteers enhanced visual reaction times. [45] Chronic caffeine intake also improves choice reaction times and tests of visual vigilance. [46] A dose of 2mg/kg enhanced reaction times in both people who did not habitually use caffeine and habitual users who had withdrawn. [47] Subjects who ingested 250mg of caffeine improved visual reaction times but did not increase their performance on a semantic reasoning test. [48] Both higher (>40mg/day) and lower (<40mg/day) habitual caffeine users experienced improvement on tests of speed in a finger tapping exercise and a choice reaction time test after two doses of caffeine (150mg and 100mg) given 75 minutes apart. [49] Administration of 100-400mg caffeine improved memory retention a day after ingestion. [50] Furthermore, doses of 100-400mg increased achievement on tasks measuring global processing. [51] In a series of twenty-four older individuals, mean 68.8, consumption of 200mg caffeine or a placebo drink half an hour before performing a memory task while undergoing functional magnetic resonance imaging revealed that caffeine augments enhancement of regions of the brain involved in working memory, especially the parietal, pre-frontal, occipital, and ventral premotor cortices , and the supplementary motor areas. [52] One study of caffeine found that the reduction velocity of cognitive processing in older individuals associated with serum acetylcholinergic activity was correlated with a serum caffeine metabolite. [53]

Beyond the potential influence of short term administration, caffeine may improve the function of elderly subjects with dementing illness. [54] Caffeine intake in the highest tertile (>62mg/day was less likely to lead to a 2 point decrement on the Mini-Mental Status Examination (MMSE) than those in the lowest tertile (<22mg/day). [55] In a cohort study of elderly persons (ages 65-88) with mild cognitive impairment (MCI), participants who eventually developed dementia had serum caffeine concentrations that were half the mean of those persons who did become demented two to four years later. [56] No subject whose concentration was below 1200ng/ml developed dementia. In another investigation of 2494 individuals, there was an association between decreased risk of ultimately developing dementia and highest quartile of caffeine use in midlife (adjust OR 0.45; 95% CI 023-0.89). [57] In a case-control study from Portugal, caffeine users were protected against development of Alzheimer's Disease (O.R. 0.40, 95% confidence interval= 0.25-0.67). [58] A metaanalysis of the relationship between caffeine intake and dementia observed a relative risk for cognitive decline of 0.84. [59] In a Scottish population cohort followed from birth to old age, there was an association between ingestion of coffee and reading test scores. [60] However, it is also possible that those with better scores preferred to drink coffee, and socioeconomic status may have confounded the results. [61]

However, there are some caveats. The form in which caffeine is ingested may make a difference. In 676 European men, those who included coffee as part of their diet experienced a 1.4 reduction in the rate of decline of cognition on the MMSE($p<0.001$). [62] Coffee (O.R 0.69 95% C.I. 0.50-0.69), but not tea consumption, correlated with dementia incidence in a study of 6434 elderly Canadians. [63] However, dose-dependent tea ingestion was inversely associated with cognitive decline in 1438 Chinese participants, initially normal over age 55 [64] Such studies have not yet been able to discriminate between the effects of dose and form of caffeine.

A gender difference may exist in the association between the consumption of caffeinated beverages and cognition. In the 4809 participant Cardiovascular Health Study, consumption of caffeinated beverages was associated with mental status exam scores in women but not men. [65] An additional investigation from France in 4197 women and 2820 men also observed a relationship between caffeine consumption and memory testing in women but not in men. [66] Women drinking more than three servings of caffeinated beverages were less likely to have white matter lesions in their brains. [67] A systematic review concluded that, in general, there was a relationship between caffeinated beverage use and cognitive preservation which was stronger for women than men. [70] However, there was less evidence for its dose-dependency.

In addition to its potential benefit on cognition, there has been preliminary investigation of a potential role for caffeine in mood disorders. An epidemiologic study of more than 50,000 women noted an association between coffee consumption and risk of depression in women. Women who drank any caffeinated coffee had a lower risk of developing depression than those who did not. [71] In 3223 individuals in a cohort from England, caffeine consumption correlated with a lower risk for depression. [72] Tea drinking was associated with a reduced incidence of depression(O.R. 0.47 ,95% CI 0.27-0.83) in 2011 Finns. [73] One investigation compared the effect of acute caffeine ingestion on mood and fatigue. [74] Ten elderly (ages 50-67) and ten younger women (ages 18-22) who were habitual caffeine consumers took a dose of 5mg/kg and completed a Profile of Mood States (POMS) questionnaire, both before and two hours after they consumed the caffeine. Depression subscale scores improved significantly in older, but not younger participants, although younger individuals observed a better tension and fatigue subscores, which older participants did not.

FUTURE DIRECTIONS AND CONCLUSION

Our knowledge of the effect of caffeine on physical performance and cognition is rudimentary. Few prospective studies have been performed on physical performance in elderly individuals, and interpretation of what little data has been obtained is confounded by the effect of caffeine dependence of subjects. No long–term use studies have been completed in older persons. Only epidemiologic studies have explored the influence of caffeine on cognition in aged individuals, and a single small study examined a potential effect on mood.

There remain many important questions for future study. One is the appropriate timing after administration to observe the desired effect. Many investigations have employed protocols in which subjects are tested sixty minutes post-ingestion since peak serum concentrations are reached then, but another hypothesis posits that maximal benefit occurs after three hours, because caffeine stimulates the breakdown of fats into free fatty acids, which peak at three hours, although this has not been proven. [75] The exact dose which should be given to subjects also requires further study. Many investigations give a fixed dose, but a dose giving a fixed concentration by body weight might be more appropriate, as used in previously mentioned study in elderly subjects. [6, 75]

Another question is which form of caffeine is optimal for maximum benefit. As caffeine can be consumed in numerous beverage forms, or a tablet, it is not clear which would be most effective in older persons. In one study, both caffeine tablets and instant coffee equally enhanced cycling times over a placebo in athletes. [76] On the other hand, a review, based on the results of studies in younger individuals in which caffeine was added to decaffeinated coffee, and in which regular coffee was compared to caffeine tablets, concluded that caffeine tablets alone was superior to coffee. [75]

Potential synergies between caffeine and naturally-occurring substances found in caffeinated beverages have also been studied. In a preliminary trial, thirty-nine normal subjects between ages 53 and 79 consumed caffeinated coffee, decaffeinated coffee, and decaffeinated coffee with extra chlorogenic acid, a polyphenol coffee constituent. [76] Caffeinated coffee improved scores, several tests of mood an attention, but the coffee with extra chlorogenic acid had similar, albeit weaker effects.

The interaction of caffeine and L-theanine, a tea constituent, has been the subject of a number of investigations. [77] In three studies, the combination of caffeine, and L-theanine improved precision and velocity on attention tests and task switching more than either component alone. [78-80] However, in another investigation, the combination did improve another measure of visual processing. [81] Theanine did not enhance a measure of alertness augmented by caffeine in an additional study. [82]

Energy drinks contain sugars and other carbohydrates that might also synergize with caffeine, and people who consume caffeine also frequently add sugars or sugar-containing substances, such as milk or cream, to their caffeinated beverages. Energy drinks have been shown to enhance performance in exercise and on athletic performance, [83, 84] but studies have not been published comparing the benefit of sugar-laden energy drinks with caffeine alone. In one trial, caffeine and glucose combined had synergistic effects on memory and attention. [85] In cyclists, the combination of caffeine and carbohydrates improved simulated racing times more than each component alone. [86]

Other influences may modify caffeine's effect. In young habitual caffeine users, expectancy impacts caffeine's augmentation of visual attention and mood. [87] In fact, maximizing the effect of caffeine in elderly individuals, as well as in young, may require greater understanding of many potential interacting influences.

REFERENCES

[1] Massey LK. Caffeine and the elderly. *Drugs Aging* 1998;13:43-50.

[2] Goldstein ER, Ziegenfuss T, Kalman D, Kreider R, Campbell B, Wilborn C, et al. International society of sports nutrition position stand: caffeine and performance. *J. Int. Soc. Sports Nutr.* 2010;7:5.

[3] Davis JK, Green JM. Caffeine and anaerobic performance: ergogenic value and mechanisms of action. *Sports Med.* 2009;39:813-32.

[4] Astorino TA, Roberson DW. Efficacy of acute caffeine ingestion for short-term high-intensity exercise performance: a systematic review. *J. Strength Cond. Res.* 2010;24:257-65.

[5] Astorino TA, Terzi MN, Roberson DW, Burnett TR. Effect of two doses of caffeine on muscular function during isokinetic exercise. *Med. Sci. Sports Exerc.* 2010;42:2205-10.

[6] Norager CB, Jensen MB, Madsen MR, Laurberg S. Caffeine improves endurance in 75-yr-old citizens: a randomized, double-blind, placebo-controlled, crossover study. *J. Appl. Physiol.* 2005;99:2302-6.

[7] Witham MD, Sugden JA, Sumukadas D, Dryburgh M, McMurdo ME. A comparison of the Endurance Shuttle Walk test and the Six Minute Walk test for assessment of exercise capacity in older people. *Aging Clin. Exp. Res.* 2012;24:176-80.

[8] Tallis J, Duncan MJ, Wright SL, Eyre EL, Bryant E, Langdon D, et al. Assessment of the ergogenic effect of caffeine supplementation on mood, anticipation timing, and muscular strength in older adults. *Physiological reports* 2013;1:e00072.

[9] Jensen MB, Norager CB, Fenger-Gron M, Weinmann A, Moller N, Madsen MR, Laurberg S Caffeine supplementation had no effect on endurance capacity in elderly subjects who had abstained from caffeine-containing nutrition for 8 hours. *J. Caffeine Res.* 2011;1:109-16.

[10] Silva-Cavalcante MD, Correia-Oliveira CR, Santos RA, Lopes-Silva JP, Lima HM, Bertuzzi R, et al. Caffeine increases anaerobic work and restores cycling performance following a protocol designed to lower endogenous carbohydrate availability. *PLoS One* 2013;8:e72025.

[11] Mohr M, Nielsen JJ, Bangsbo J. Caffeine intake improves intense intermittent exercise performance and reduces muscle interstitial potassium accumulation. *J. Appl. Physiol.* (1985) 2011;111:1372-9.

[12] Kalmar JM, Cafarelli E. Caffeine: a valuable tool to study central fatigue in humans? *Exerc. Sport Sci. Rev.* 2004;32:143-7.

[13] Bazzucchi I, Felici F, Montini M, Figura F, Sacchetti M. Caffeine improves neuromuscular function during maximal dynamic exercise. *Muscle Nerve* 2011;43:839-44.

[14] Corsetti G, Pasini E, Assanelli D, Saligari E, Adobati M, Bianchi R. Acute caffeine administration decreased NOS and Bcl2 expression in rat skeletal muscles. *Pharmacol. Res.* 2007;55:96-103.

[15] Corsetti G, Pasini E, Assanelli D, Bianchi R. Effects of acute caffeine administration on NOS and Bax/Bcl2 expression in the myocardium of rat. *Pharmacol. Res.* 2008;57:19-25.

[16] Duncan MJ, Stanley M, Parkhouse N, Cook K, Smith M. Acute caffeine ingestion enhances strength performance and reduces perceived exertion and muscle pain perception during resistance exercise. *European journal of sport science* 2013;13:392-9.

[17] Maridakis V, O'Connor PJ, Dudley GA, McCully KK. Caffeine attenuates delayed-onset muscle pain and force loss following eccentric exercise. *The journal of pain: official journal of the American Pain Society* 2007;8:237-43.

[18] Astorino TA, Cottrell T, Talhami Lozano A, Aburto-Pratt K, Duhon J. Effect of caffeine on RPE and perceptions of pain, arousal, and pleasure/displeasure during a cycling time trial in endurance trained and active men. *Physiol. Behav.* 2012;106:211-7.

[19] Astorino TA, Roupoli LR, Valdivieso BR. Caffeine does not alter RPE or pain perception during intense exercise in active women. *Appetite* 2012;59:585-90.

[20] Killen LG, Green JM, O'Neal EK, McIntosh JR, Hornsby J, Coates TE. Effects of caffeine on session ratings of perceived exertion. *Eur. J. Appl. Physiol.* 2013;113:721-7.

[21] Nehlig A. Is caffeine a cognitive enhancer? *J. Alzheimers Dis.* 2010;20 Suppl 1:S85-94.

[22] Porciuncula LO, Sallaberry C, Mioranzza S, Botton PH, Rosemberg DB. The Janus face of caffeine. *Neurochem. Int.* 2013;63:594-609.

[23] Abreu RV, Silva-Oliveira EM, Moraes MF, Pereira GS, Moraes-Santos T. Chronic coffee and caffeine ingestion effects on the cognitive function and antioxidant system of rat brains. *Pharmacol. Biochem. Behav.* 2011;99:659-64.

[24] Espinosa J, Rocha A, Nunes F, Costa MS, Schein V, Kazlauckas V, et al. Caffeine consumption prevents memory impairment, neuronal damage, and adenosine A2A receptors upregulation in the hippocampus of a rat model of sporadic dementia. *J. Alzheimers Dis.* 2013;34:509-18.

[25] Higgins GA, Grzelak ME, Pond AJ, Cohen-Williams ME, Hodgson RA, Varty GB. The effect of caffeine to increase reaction time in the rat during a test of attention is mediated through antagonism of adenosine A2A receptors. *Behav. Brain Res.* 2007;185:32-42.

[26] Chu YF, Chang WH, Black RM, Liu JR, Sompol P, Chen Y, et al. Crude caffeine reduces memory impairment and amyloid beta(1-42) levels in an Alzheimer's mouse model. *Food Chem.* 2012;135:2095-102.

[27] Prediger RD, Batista LC, Takahashi RN. Caffeine reverses age-related deficits in olfactory discrimination and social recognition memory in rats. Involvement of adenosine A1 and A2A receptors. *Neurobiol. Aging* 2005;26:957-64.

[28] Dall'Igna OP, Porciuncula LO, Souza DO, Cunha RA, Lara DR. Neuroprotection by caffeine and adenosine A2A receptor blockade of beta-amyloid neurotoxicity. *Br. J. Pharmacol.* 2003;138:1207-9.

[29] Dall'Igna OP, Fett P, Gomes MW, Souza DO, Cunha RA, Lara DR. Caffeine and adenosine A(2a) receptor antagonists prevent beta-amyloid (25-35)-induced cognitive deficits in mice. *Exp. Neurol.* 2007;203: 241-5.

[30] Arendash GW, Schleif W, Rezai-Zadeh K, Jackson EK, Zacharia LC, Cracchiolo JR, et al. Caffeine protects Alzheimer's mice against

cognitive impairment and reduces brain beta-amyloid production. *Neuroscience* 2006;142:941-52.

[31] Arendash GW, Mori T, Cao C, Mamcarz M, Runfeldt M, Dickson A, et al. Caffeine reverses cognitive impairment and decreases brain amyloid-beta levels in aged Alzheimer's disease mice. *J. Alzheimers Dis.* 2009; 17:661-80.

[32] Alzoubi KH, Abdul-Razzak KK, Khabour OF, Al-Tuweiq GM, Alzubi MA, Alkadhi KA. Caffeine prevents cognitive impairment induced by chronic psychosocial stress and/or high fat-high carbohydrate diet. *Behav. Brain Res.* 2013;237:7-14.

[33] Vila-Luna S, Cabrera-Isidoro S, Vila-Luna L, Juarez-Diaz I, Bata-Garcia JL, Alvarez-Cervera FJ, et al. Chronic caffeine consumption prevents cognitive decline from young to middle age in rats, and is associated with increased length, branching, and spine density of basal dendrites in CA1 hippocampal neurons. *Neuroscience* 2012;202:384-95.

[34] Costa MS, Botton PH, Mioranzza S, Souza DO, Porciuncula LO. Caffeine prevents age-associated recognition memory decline and changes brain-derived neurotrophic factor and tirosine kinase receptor (TrkB) content in mice. *Neuroscience* 2008;153:1071-8.

[35] Costa MS, Botton PH, Mioranzza S, Ardais AP, Moreira JD, Souza DO, et al. Caffeine improves adult mice performance in the object recognition task and increases BDNF and TrkB independent on phospho-CREB immunocontent in the hippocampus. *Neurochem. Int.* 2008;53:89-94.

[36] Dragicevic N, Delic V, Cao C, Copes N, Lin X, Mamcarz M, et al. Caffeine increases mitochondrial function and blocks melatonin signaling to mitochondria in Alzheimer's mice and cells. *Neuropharmacology* 2012;63:1368-79.

[37] Prasanthi JR, Dasari B, Marwarha G, Larson T, Chen X, Geiger JD, et al. Caffeine protects against oxidative stress and Alzheimer's disease-like pathology in rabbit hippocampus induced by cholesterol-enriched diet. *Free Radic. Biol. Med.* 2010;49:1212-20.

[38] Wostyn P, Van Dam D, Audenaert K, De Deyn PP. Increased Cerebrospinal Fluid Production as a Possible Mechanism Underlying Caffeine's Protective Effect against Alzheimer's Disease. *International journal of Alzheimer's disease* 2011;2011:617420.

[39] Chen X, Ghribi O, Geiger JD. Caffeine protects against disruptions of the blood-brain barrier in animal models of Alzheimer's and Parkinson's diseases. *J. Alzheimers Dis.* 2010;20 Suppl 1:S127-41.

[40] Chen X, Gawryluk JW, Wagener JF, Ghribi O, Geiger JD. Caffeine blocks disruption of blood brain barrier in a rabbit model of Alzheimer's disease. *J. Neuroinflammation* 2008;5:12.

[41] Chen X, Lan X, Roche I, Liu R, Geiger JD. Caffeine protects against MPTP-induced blood-brain barrier dysfunction in mouse striatum. *J. Neurochem.* 2008;107:1147-57.

[42] Alhaider IA, Aleisa AM, Tran TT, Alzoubi KH, Alkadhi KA. Chronic caffeine treatment prevents sleep deprivation-induced impairment of cognitive function and synaptic plasticity. *Sleep* 2010;33:437-44.

[43] Marques S, Batalha VL, Lopes LV, Outeiro TF. Modulating Alzheimer's disease through caffeine: a putative link to epigenetics. *J. Alzheimers Dis.* 2011;24 Suppl 2:161-71.

[44] Olson CA, Thornton JA, Adam GE, Lieberman HR. Effects of 2 adenosine antagonists, quercetin and caffeine, on vigilance and mood. *J. Clin. Psychopharmacol.* 2010;30:573-8.

[45] Beaven CM, Ekstrom J. A comparison of blue light and caffeine effects on cognitive function and alertness in humans. *PLoS One* 2013; 8:e76707.

[46] Judelson DA, Armstrong LE, Sokmen B, Roti MW, Casa DJ, Kellogg MD. Effect of chronic caffeine intake on choice reaction time, mood, and visual vigilance. *Physiol. Behav.* 2005;85:629-34.

[47] Smith AP, Christopher G, Sutherland D. Acute effects of caffeine on attention: a comparison of non-consumers and withdrawn consumers. *J. Psychopharmacol.* 2013;27:77-83.

[48] Attwood A, Terry P, Higgs S. Conditioned effects of caffeine on performance in humans. *Physiol. Behav.* 2010;99:286-93.

[49] Rogers PJ, Heatherley SV, Mullings EL, Smith JE. Faster but not smarter: effects of caffeine and caffeine withdrawal on alertness and performance. *Psychopharmacology* (Berl) 2013;226:229-40.

[50] Borota D, Murray E, Keceli G, Chang A, Watabe JM, Ly M, et al. Post-study caffeine administration enhances memory consolidation in humans. *Nat. Neurosci.* 2014;17:201-3.

[51] Mahoney CR, Brunye TT, Giles G, Lieberman HR, Taylor HA. Caffeine-induced physiological arousal accentuates global processing biases. *Pharmacol. Biochem. Behav.* 2011;99:59-65.

[52] Haller S, Rodriguez C, Moser D, Toma S, Hofmeister J, Sinanaj I, et al. Acute caffeine administration impact on working memory-related brain activation and functional connectivity in the elderly: a BOLD and perfusion MRI study. *Neuroscience* 2013;250:364-71.

[53] Nebes RD, Pollock BG, Halligan EM, Houck P, Saxton JA. Cognitive slowing associated with elevated serum anticholinergic activity in older individuals is decreased by caffeine use. *Am. J. Geriatr. Psychiatry* 2011;19:169-75.

[54] Eskelinen MH, Kivipelto M. Caffeine as a protective factor in dementia and Alzheimer's disease. *J. Alzheimers Dis.* 2010;20 Suppl 1:S167-74.

[55] Santos C, Lunet N, Azevedo A, de Mendonca A, Ritchie K, Barros H. Caffeine intake is associated with a lower risk of cognitive decline: a cohort study from Portugal. *J. Alzheimers Dis.* 2010;20 Suppl 1:S175-85.

[56] Cao C, Loewenstein DA, Lin X, Zhang C, Wang L, Duara R, et al. High Blood caffeine levels in MCI linked to lack of progression to dementia. *J. Alzheimers Dis.* 2012;30:559-72.

[57] Gelber RP, Petrovitch H, Masaki KH, Ross GW, White LR. Coffee intake in midlife and risk of dementia and its neuropathologic correlates. *J. Alzheimers Dis.* 2011;23:607-15.

[58] Maia L, de Mendonca A. Does caffeine intake protect from Alzheimer's disease? *Eur. J. Neurol.* 2002;9:377-82.

[59] Santos C, Costa J, Santos J, Vaz-Carneiro A, Lunet N. Caffeine intake and dementia: systematic review and meta-analysis. *J. Alzheimers Dis.* 2010;20 Suppl 1:S187-204.

[60] Corley J, Jia X, Kyle JA, Gow AJ, Brett CE, Starr JM, et al. Caffeine consumption and cognitive function at age 70: the Lothian Birth Cohort 1936 study. *Psychosom. Med*;72:206-14.

[61] Kyle J, Fox HC, Whalley LJ. Caffeine, cognition, and socioeconomic status. *J. Alzheimers Dis.* 2010;20 Suppl 1:S151-9.

[62] van Gelder BM, Buijsse B, Tijhuis M, Kalmijn S, Giampaoli S, Nissinen A, et al. Coffee consumption is inversely associated with cognitive decline in elderly European men: the FINE Study. *Eur. J. Clin. Nutr.* 2007;61:226-32.

[63] Lindsay J, Laurin D, Verreault R, Hebert R, Helliwell B, Hill GB, et al. Risk factors for Alzheimer's disease: a prospective analysis from the Canadian Study of Health and Aging. *Am. J. Epidemiol.* 2002;156:445-53.

[64] Ng TP, Feng L, Niti M, Kua EH, Yap KB. Tea consumption and cognitive impairment and decline in older Chinese adults. *Am. J. Clin. Nutr.* 2008;88:224-31.

[65] Arab L, Biggs ML, O'Meara ES, Longstreth WT, Crane PK, Fitzpatrick AL. Gender differences in tea, coffee, and cognitive decline in the

elderly: the Cardiovascular Health Study. *J. Alzheimers Dis.* 2011; 27:553-66.

[66] Ritchie K, Carriere I, de Mendonca A, Portet F, Dartigues JF, Rouaud O, et al. The neuroprotective effects of caffeine: a prospective population study (the Three City Study). *Neurology* 2007;69:536-45.

[67] Ritchie K, Artero S, Portet F, Brickman A, Muraskin J, Beanino E, et al. Caffeine, cognitive functioning, and white matter lesions in the elderly: establishing causality from epidemiological evidence. *J. Alzheimers Dis.* 2010;20 Suppl 1:S161-6.

[68] Dai Q, Borenstein AR, Wu Y, Jackson JC, Larson EB. Fruit and vegetable juices and Alzheimer's disease: the Kame Project. *Am. J. Med.* 2006;119:751-9.

[69] Laitala VS, Kaprio J, Koskenvuo M, Raiha I, Rinne JO, Silventoinen K. Coffee drinking in middle age is not associated with cognitive performance in old age. *Am. J. Clin. Nutr.* 2009;90:640-6.

[70] Arab L, Khan F, Lam H. Epidemiologic evidence of a relationship between tea, coffee, or caffeine consumption and cognitive decline. *Advances in nutrition* 2013;4:115-22.

[71] Lucas M, Mirzaei F, Pan A, Okereke OI, Willett WC, O'Reilly EJ, et al. Coffee, caffeine, and risk of depression among women. *Arch. Intern. Med.* 2011;171:1571-8.

[72] Smith AP. Caffeine, cognitive failures and health in a non-working community sample. *Hum. Psychopharmacol.* 2009;24:29-34.

[73] Hintikka J, Tolmunen T, Honkalampi K, Haatainen K, Koivumaa-Honkanen H, Tanskanen A, et al. Daily tea drinking is associated with a low level of depressive symptoms in the Finnish general population. *Eur. J. Epidemiol.* 2005;20:359-63.

[74] Arciero PJ, Ormsbee MJ. Relationship of blood pressure, behavioral mood state, and physical activity following caffeine ingestion in younger and older women. *Appl. Physiol. Nutr. Metab.* 2009;34:754-62.

[75] Graham TE. Caffeine and exercise: metabolism, endurance and performance. *Sports Med.* 2001;31:785-807.

[76] Hodgson AB, Randell RK, Jeukendrup AE. The metabolic and performance effects of caffeine compared to coffee during endurance exercise. *PLoS One* 2013;8:e59561.

[77] Bryan J. Psychological effects of dietary components of tea: caffeine and L-theanine. *Nutr. Rev.* 2008;66:82-90.

[78] Owen GN, Parnell H, De Bruin EA, Rycroft JA. The combined effects of L-theanine and caffeine on cognitive performance and mood. *Nutr. Neurosci.* 2008;11:193-8.

[79] Giesbrecht T, Rycroft JA, Rowson MJ, De Bruin EA. The combination of L-theanine and caffeine improves cognitive performance and increases subjective alertness. *Nutr. Neurosci.* 2010;13:283-90.

[80] Einother SJ, Martens VE, Rycroft JA, De Bruin EA. L-theanine and caffeine improve task switching but not intersensory attention or subjective alertness. *Appetite* 2010;54:406-9.

[81] Haskell CF, Kennedy DO, Milne AL, Wesnes KA, Scholey AB. The effects of L-theanine, caffeine and their combination on cognition and mood. *Biol. Psychol.* 2008;77:113-22.

[82] Rogers PJ, Smith JE, Heatherley SV, Pleydell-Pearce CW. Time for tea: mood, blood pressure and cognitive performance effects of caffeine and theanine administered alone and together. *Psychopharmacology* (Berl) 2008;195:569-77.

[83] Del Coso J, Munoz-Fernandez VE, Munoz G, Fernandez-Elias VE, Ortega JF, Hamouti N, et al. Effects of a caffeine-containing energy drink on simulated soccer performance. *PLoS One* 2012;7:e31380.

[84] Del Coso J, Salinero JJ, Gonzalez-Millan C, Abian-Vicen J, Perez-Gonzalez B. Dose response effects of a caffeine-containing energy drink on muscle performance: a repeated measures design. *J. Int. Soc. Sports Nutr.* 2012;9:21.

[85] Adan A, Serra-Grabulosa JM. Effects of caffeine and glucose, alone and combined, on cognitive performance. *Hum. Psychopharmacol.* 2010; 25:310-7.

[86] Acker-Hewitt TL, Shafer BM, Saunders MJ, Goh Q, Luden ND. Independent and combined effects of carbohydrate and caffeine ingestion on aerobic cycling performance in the fed state. *Appl. Physiol. Nutr. Metab.* 2012;37:276-83.

[87] Elliman NA, Ash J, Green MW. Pre-existent expectancy effects in the relationship between caffeine and performance. *Appetite* 2010;55:355-8.

In: Caffeine
Editor: Aimée S. Tolley

ISBN: 978-1-63117-777-4
© 2014 Nova Science Publishers, Inc.

Chapter 2

CAFFEINE FACILITATES CONDITIONED OPERANT RESPONSES ASSOCIATED WITH SELF-ADMINISTRATION OF HIGH FAT FOODS IN RATS

Xiu Liu[*]

Department of Psychiatry and Human Behavior,
University of Mississippi Medical Center, Jackson, MS, US

ABSTRACT

In light of the fact that our previous research showed that caffeine facilitated the behavioral motivation effect of an environmental cue conditioned to nicotine self-administration (Liu and Jernigan 2012), the present study was designed to examine the issue of whether the enhancing effect of caffeine on conditioned reinforcement extends to behavior supported by a cue previously conditioned to a natural reward food. Male Sprague-Dawley rats, satiated with standard laboratory chow, were trained to self-administer food pellets containing high fat contents on a progressive ratio schedule of reinforcement. Each pellet delivery was associated with a sensory stimulus so that the later acquired incentive value and become a food-conditioned cue. After lever responses were

---

[*] Corresponding Author: Xiu Liu, MD, PhD, Associate Professor, Department of Psychiatry and Human Behavior, University of Mississippi Medical Center, 2500 North State Street, Jackson, MS 39216, Tel: (601) 984-2875, Fax: (601) 984-5889, Email: xliu@umc.edu.

extinguished by withholding food pellet and its cue, effects of caffeine (5 mg/kg, i.p.) administration alone or together with re-presentation of food cue on lever responses were examined in the test sessions where responses did not result in delivery of food pellets. Re-presentations of the food cue effectively reinstated extinguished responses on the previously active, food-reinforced lever. Although pre-session administration of caffeine on its own did not increase responses, caffeine significantly potentiated the cue-induced reinstatement of food-seeking responses. These data demonstrate that acute caffeine administration can facilitate the behavioral motivation effect of natural reward (food) conditioned stimuli. This finding suggests that caffeine consumption may heighten food-seeking behavior triggered by exposure to the food-associated environmental stimuli.

Keywords: Caffeine, conditioned stimuli, extinction, food, food-seeking, rats, reinstatement, self-administration

INTRODUCTION

Caffeine is the most popularly consumed psychoactive substance all over the world (Glade 2010). It can be found in foods and drinks as well as many over-the-counter medications. In the United States, majority of the adults report regular caffeine use, mostly from coffee (70%), soda (16%), and tea (12%) (Frary et al. 2005). A recently emerging source of caffeine is the energy drink, which contains 50-505 mg caffeine per can or bottle (Aranda and Morlock 2006). The energy drink market has grown exponentially, with approximately 200 new brands launched in the United States during the 1-year period ending July 2007 (Packaged-Facts 2007). This fast-growing energy drink market will expose even more people to caffeine.

There have been some studies reporting that caffeine produces an effect on appetite. In humans, for example, caffeine appeared to have a small reducing effect on eating and caloric intake (Comer et al. 1997; Tremblay et al. 1988) and amplified the attenuating effect of nicotine on appetite (Jessen et al. 2005). In animal research, in contrast, studies have showed inconsistent results, from a suppressant effect of caffeine treatment on food intake and body weight gain to lack of a significant effect in rats (Pettenuzzo et al. 2008; Racotta et al. 1994). In an earlier report, caffeine decreased operant lever press responses for food rewards (Carney 1982). Therefore, it is yet still controversial on the issue of whether caffeine exerts a direct anorectic effect.

Although the psychoactive effects of caffeine are moderate relative to other prototypical stimulants such as cocaine and amphetamine (Antoniou et al. 1998; Wood et al. 2014), caffeine increases attention and vigilance (Boutrel and Koob 2004; Brunye et al. 2010; Caballero et al. 2011). Caffeine has been found to effectively reinstate cocaine-seeking responses using an extinction-reinstatement procedure in animals (Schenk and Partridge 1999; Schenk et al. 1996; Worley et al. 1994). Our recent work demonstrated that acute caffeine administration, albeit did not on its own reinstate lever responses in caffeine naïve rats, significantly enhanced the conditioned behavioral motivation by a nicotine cue (Liu and Jernigan 2012). Based on this line of research, we hypothesized that the facilitating effects of acute caffeine exposure on conditioned motivation may extend to responses supported by cues previously conditioned to self-administration of natural rewards such as food.

This study was designed, using an extinction-reinstatement paradigm, to examine whether caffeine administration on its own motivates food-seeking responses and/or interact with food-conditioned cue and thereby facilitates the cue-induced reinstatement of food-seeking behavior. Specifically, caffeine was intraperitoneally administered before the reinstatement test sessions that were performed immediately after food-maintained lever responding was extinguished. The caffeine dose used was 5 mg/kg, which was selected based on the following facts: (1) Moderate per capita daily intake of caffeine in humans is approximately 280 mg, which is equivalent to 4-5 mg/kg, whereas intake over 700 mg/day or 10 mg/kg is considered heavy caffeine consumption or sometimes referred to "caffeinism." (2) Pretreatment with caffeine up to 5 mg/kg produced no change in operant responses for other psycostimulants such as nicotine self-administration or the discriminative-stimulus effects of nicotine (Perkins et al. 2005). (3) Caffeine at 5 mg/kg in rats did not alter locomotor activity (Antoniou et al. 1998; Rezvani et al. 2013).

MATERIALS AND METHODS

Animals

Male Sprague-Dawley rats (Charles River, Portage, MI), 201-225 g upon arrival, were used. The animals were individually housed in a humidity- and temperature-controlled (21-22°C) colony room maintained on a 12 h/12 h reversed light/dark cycle with the lights off at 8:00 AM. In the first week after arrival, rats were allowed to acclimate to the new environment and daily handling. The rats had unlimited access to water and standard laboratory rat chow except a brief period of food restriction for lever-press training as described below. Experimental sessions were conducted during the dark phase at the same time each day (9:00 AM-3:00 PM). All of the experimental procedures were performed in accordance with the National Institutes of Health *Guide for the Care and Use of Laboratory Animals* and approved by the University of Mississippi Medical Center Institutional Animal Care and Use Committee.

Experimental Apparatus

Standard operant conditioning chambers located inside sound-attenuating, ventilated cubicles (Med Associates, St. Albans, VT) were used. The chambers were equipped with two retractable response levers on one side panel, a 28-V white light above each lever, and a red chamber light on upper center of the opposite panel. Between the two levers was a food pellet trough. Experimental events and data collection were automatically controlled and recorded by a Med Associates interfaced computer and software (Med-PC version IV).

Lever-Press Training

After one week of acclimation, rats were placed on a food restriction regimen with 20 g chow/day in order to facilitate the learning of operant responding for food reward. In the daily training sessions, rats were placed in the experimental chambers and the sessions started with introduction of one lever. Responding on the lever was rewarded with the delivery of a food pellet (45 mg) on a fixed-ratio (FR) 1 schedule of reinforcement. The sessions lasted 1 hour and rats could earn at maximum 45 food pellets in a single session. After the rats learned to respond, the reinforcement schedule was increased to FR5. The training sessions finished once rats earned 45 food pellets on the FR5 schedule in a single session. Successful lever-press training was achieved within 2-5 sessions. Thus, food restriction regimen lasted at most for 5 days. After the lever press training and throughout the following experiments, rats had free access to chow in their home cages.

Self-Administration and Conditioning

After lever-press training, rats were subject to daily 1-h food self-administration sessions. The experimental sessions started with introduction of the two levers and illumination of the red chamber light. Responses on the active level were reinforced with delivery of high fat food pellets (Bio-Serv, Frenchtown, NJ). The pellets contained 35% fatty contents relative to 5.5% fat of the nutritionally balanced, standard laboratory chow. In general, there were to some extent differences in the taste and palatability between the standard chow and high-fat food pellets with the later being more palatable for rats. For the purpose of measuring rats' motivation for obtaining the high fat food reward and limiting the total number of pellets earned, a progressive-ratio (PR) schedule of reinforcement was used. The PR schedule was modified from the formula $5e^{(0.2 \times \text{infusion number})-5}$ (Depoortere et al. 1993) so that the response requirement for successive food pellet delivery was 3, 6, 10, 15, 20, 25, 32, 40, 50, 62, 77, 95, 118, 145, 179, 219, 268, and so on. Each food pellet delivery was signaled with the presentation of a stimulus consisting of 5 s tone and 20 s turn-on of the light above the active lever. As such, the stimulus was established as a conditioned stimulus or cue. Following each delivery of reinforcer, there was a 20 s timeout period, during which time the active lever responses resulted in no consequence but were recorded. Throughout the experiments, responses on the second, inactive lever did not produce any programmed consequence. To establish steady food self-administration behavior and equalize experience in lever press for food reward, all rats received 20 sessions.

Extinction

After completion of self-administration and conditioning phase, rats were subjected to daily extinction sessions. Lever responding was extinguished by withholding food pellets and associated cue presentation. In these extinction sessions, responses on the previously active lever did not resulted in any programmed consequence. The criterion for extinction was three consecutive sessions in which the number of active lever responses per session was ≤20% of the average across the last three self-administration sessions. To habituate rats to the intraperitoneal administration procedure and eliminate possible effects of injection stress on operant behavior, rats received an intraperitonal administration of 1 ml/kg saline 5 min before extinction sessions for three days.

Reinstatement Tests

The reinstatement tests began 1 day after the final extinction session. As happened in the self-administration and conditioning as well as extinction phases, the test session started with introduction of the two levers and illumination of the red chamber light. Although there was still no delivery of food pellets in the test sessions, whether responses on the active lever resulted in re-presentation of food cue was dependent on the test conditions described below. Responses on the inactive lever had no consequence. The test sessions lasted 1 hour.

Effects of Caffeine, Food Cue, and Their Combination on the Reinstatement of Food Seeking

In ten rats, three reinstatement test sessions were conducted in the following order: (1) with the pre-session caffeine but without food cue presentation, (2) with response-contingent presentation of food cue but without pre-session caffeine, and (3) with both pre-session caffeine and food cue.

Specifically, to test whether caffeine alone could reinstate food-seeking responses, rats were subjected to an intraperitoneal administration of caffeine at 5 mg/kg (1 ml/kg in volume) 5 min prior to the test session. During the session, responses on the active lever did not produce any programmed consequence. To test whether representation of food cue alone could reinstate food-seeking responses, rats were subjected to an intraperitoneal administration of vehicle saline at 1 ml/kg volume 5 min prior to the test session. To inform the rats of the availability of the food cue, a single response-noncontingent cue was presented together with start of the test session. Then throughout the test session, responses on the active lever resulted in representation of the cue on a FR5 schedule with the 20 s timeout period in effect. To test effects of the combination of caffeine and food cue, rats were subjected to an intraperitoneal administration of caffeine at 5 mg/kg 5 min prior to the test, Then, a single presentation of response-noncontingent cue was given together with start of the session, and during the session responses on the active lever resulted in representation of the cue on a FR5 schedule with the 20 s timeout period in effect. To guarantee the extinction baseline before each test session, two extinction sessions were inserted between the three reinstatement tests.

Data Analysis

The data are expressed as the mean±SEM number of lever responses, breaking points of active lever responses, and food pellets earned. A one-way analysis of variance (ANOVA) with repeated measures was used to analyze the data obtained from the reinstatement test sessions. Then, Newman-Keuls *post hoc* tests were used to verify differences among individual means.

RESULTS

Food Self-administration and Conditioning

Rats developed in the daily 1-h sessions stable level of lever press responses for food self-administration under the PR schedule of reinforcement. In summary, averaged across the final three sessions (sessions 18, 19, and 20), the rats made an effort of emitting about 158 response on the active lever in order to earn the delivery of food pellets containing high fat contents.

Table 1. Behavioral profile of rats (n=10) that self-administered high fat food pellets under a PR schedule of reinforcement

	Mean±SEM
Self-administration	
Active lever responses	158±20
Braking points of active lever responses	44±4
Inactive lever responses	10±2
Food pellets earned	7±0.5
Extinction	
Active lever responses	25±3
Inactive lever responses	5±1

These animals were provided free access to standard laboratory rat chow in their home cages. Data are expressed as the average across the final three sessions of both the self-administration and extinction phases.

These animals showed significant level of motivation for the procurement of high fat food rewards even though they were satiated with standard laboratory chow in their home cages. It could be reflected by the final and highest number (44±4) of lever responses rats made for getting a single food pellet delivery, defined as the breaking point. These rats earned 7±0.5 deliveries of high fat food pellets. That meant that in each session the rats acquired about seven pairings of the stimulus cue with food pellet delivery. In contrast, responses on the inactive, non-rewarded lever remained at very low level. Detailed data are presented in Table 1.

Extinction of Food-Reinforced Lever Responses

In the first extinction session, rats emitted a mean±SEM of 166±23 responses on the previously active and food-reinforced lever. This number was slightly higher than the averaged responses of the last three self-administration sessions as shown in Table 1. However, in the subsequent daily extinction sessions, lever responses decreased dramatically. A one-way ANOVA with repeated measures on the number of active lever responses showed a significant main effect of sessions [$F(9,81)=14.32$, $p=0.0001$]. It meant that withholding the delivery of food pellets and its associated presentation of the cue extinguished lever responses. All rats reached the extinction criterion within 10 daily extinction sessions. Detailed data are shown in Table 1.

Effects of Caffeine, Food Cues, and Their Combination on Food-seeking Responses

After lever responses were extinguished, the reinstatement test sessions are conducted under three different conditions. As shown in Figure 1, pre-session caffeine administration did not reinstate extinguished lever responding. That is, the responses on the previously food reinforced active lever remained at a low level similar to the extinction baseline. However, as expected, re-presentation of the food cue effectively reinstated active lever responses, indicating the conditioned incentive properties of the food cue. Interestingly, pre-session caffeine administration significantly enhanced the effect of food cues in the pre-session caffeine plus cue condition, leading to a higher level of food-seeking responses.

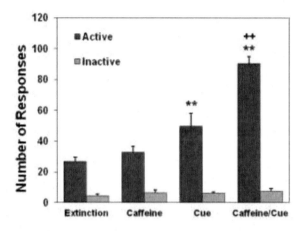

Figure 1. Lever responses in the reinstatement tests in rats (n=10). *Caffeine* represents a test condition under which rats received a pre-session caffeine administration but without cue presentation during the session. *Cue* represents a test condition under which active lever responses resulted in re-presentation of the food cue after rats received a pre-session administration of saline. *Caffeine/Cue* represents the test condition combining pre-session caffeine administration and in-session cue presentation. The data are expressed as mean±SEM lever responses. *$p<0.05$, **$p<0.01$, significant difference from extinction condition. ++$p<0.01$, significant difference from either caffeine or cue condition.

One-way ANOVA of the active lever responses revealed a significant effect of test condition [$F(3,27)=45.24$, $p=0.0001$]. Subsequent Newman-Keuls *post hoc* tests verified a significant difference ($p<0.01$) in the number of active lever responses under the cue condition and pre-session caffeine plus cue condition compared to the extinction baseline and pre-session caffeine conditions as well as pre-session caffeine plus cue condition compared to pre-session caffeine and cue conditions. However, responses on the inactive lever remained at low levels that were indistinguishable among conditions.

DISCUSSION

This study used an extinction and reinstatement procedure to investigate effects of caffeine administration on food-seeking behavior. The main findings were that although pre-session administration of caffeine at 5 mg/kg on its own did not change operant behavior it significantly enhanced the behavioral motivation effect of a cue conditioned to the intake of foods containing high fat contents. The data suggest that caffeine consumption may contribute to heightened food-seeking behavior associated with exposure to the environmental stimuli previously conditioned to eating fatty foods.

Due to the fact that caffeine is a psychomotor stimulant that produces locomotor activation (Bedingfield et al. 1998; Garrett and Holtzman 1994), a convenient explanation for the present data is speculated. That is, the ability of caffeine to enhance the response-reinstating effect of the food cue may be attributable to general arousal and/or motor activation by caffeine. Therefore, to properly interpret the results, the issue of whether the effects of caffeine observed in this study resulted from general arousal or locomotor activation by caffeine needs to be addressed. There were several facts that deserve our attention. First, pre-session caffeine administration by itself without presence of the food cue did not facilitate lever responses; Second, caffeine did not change responding on a reference and inactive lever under all test conditions. Third, the lack of direct activating effects of 5 mg/kg caffeine on locomotor activity is consistent with other studies. For example, our previous work showed that pre-session administration of 5 mg/kg caffeine neither changed lever press responses for intravenous self-administration of nicotine nor reinstated nicotine-seeking behavior in caffeine naïve rats although it could serve as a discriminative stimulus to enhance cue-induced nicotine seeking (Liu and Jernigan 2012). Moreover, in a variety of behavioral test paradigms including direct measurement of locomotor activity in rodents, caffeine at 5 mg/kg did not stimulate locomotor activity and the minimum dose that enhanced locomotor activity was ≥10-20 mg/kg (Antoniou et al. 1998; Cohen et al. 1991; Garrett and Holtzman 1994; Halldner et al. 2004; Jaszyna et al. 1998; Marin et al. 2011; Rezvani et al. 2013). Taken together, the behavioral effects of caffeine observed in this study were unlikely to be interpreted as a result of general arousal and/or motor activation by caffeine.

Response-contingent re-presentation of the food-conditioned cue after extinction effectively reinstated the extinguished responses on the previously food-reinforced lever, indicating the conditioned incentive properties of the cue. This result is consistent with other studies showing the behavioral motivation by food-conditioned cues (Ball et al. 2011; Floresco et al. 2008; Guy et al. 2011; Uslaner et al. 2010). It was interesting to note that pre-session administration of caffeine at 5 mg/kg significantly enhanced the behavioral motivation effect of the food cue. This finding is similar to the data obtained with a different psychostimulant, nicotine. Uslaner et al. (Uslaner et al. 2010) reported that nicotine facilitated the cue-reinstated responses on a previously sucrose-reinforced lever. The issue of whether such a facilitating effect of caffeine and nicotine can be extended to other classes of psychoactive stimulants remains to be determined. Nevertheless, the present finding is of highly clinical relevance. In human, heavy caffeine consumption or sometimes referred to "caffeinism" refers to intake of caffeine over 10 mg/kg. Moderate per capita daily intake of caffeine is approximately 4-5 mg/kg (280 mg in subjects weighing 70 kg), which corresponds to about 1-1.5 cups of coffee (Fredholm et al. 1999). As such, the observed results of this study may readily be applied to regular social coffee drinkers.

The finding that caffeine challenge alone did not reinstate extinguished food-seeking responses is in line with our previous research with nicotine (Liu and Jernigan 2012). That study used a similar experimental procedure to train rats to self-administer nicotine (0.03 mg/kg/infusion, free base). After lever responding was extinguished by withholding nicotine and its associated cue, lever press responses were examined after an intraperitoneal administration of caffeine at 5 mg/kg. The pre-session caffeine did not enhance responses on the previously active and nicotine-reinforced lever, indicating a lack of response-reinstating effect of caffeine in those nicotine trained rats. However, it is worthy to note that caffeine in the rats that had been trained to self-administer nicotine with pre-session administration of caffeine effectively reinstated extinguished nicotine-seeking behavior. In that case, pre-session caffeine was postulated to reinstate nicotine-seeking responses via its discriminative-stimulus properties. Such an occasion-setting effect of caffeine would have been more consolidated after extinction. During the extinction (i.e., saline substitution) sessions in which nicotine delivery and its associated cues were withheld, the chamber context in the absence of caffeine set an occasion for the lack of nicotine availability. As such, the self-administration and extinction sequence, albeit unlike standard discrimination training procedures, established pre-session caffeine as a discriminative stimulus. Such an account is consistent with previous studies in which discriminative stimuli effectively reinstated extinguished drug-seeking behavior in animals trained to self-administer cocaine, heroin, ethanol, nicotine, and sucrose (Alvarez-Jaimes et al. 2008; Burbassi and Cervo 2008; Ciccocioppo et al. 2001; Gracy et al. 2000; Katner et al. 1999; Wing and Shoaib 2008).

The lack of a priming effect of caffeine on food-seeking behavior observed in the present study contrasts with the results obtained from cocaine-trained rats in which a caffeine priming injection reinstated cocaine seeking (Green and Schenk 2002; Kuzmin et al. 1999; Schenk and Partridge 1999; Schenk et al. 1996; Worley et al. 1994). Two factors may underlie this discrepancy. The first is the different classes of primary rewards used (i.e., high fat food pellets and cocaine). The second is the substantial difference in the test procedures because those cocaine studies tested the effect of caffeine using a so-called within-session paradigm in which the extinction and reinstatement tests were conducted in a single session. Taken together, these research results call for future investigation on the issue of whether acute caffeine exposure produces differential effects in the abstinent subjects that used to take cocaine or natural rewards such as high fat foods.

Caffeine exerts its actions via directly antagonizing the A_1 and A_{2A} subtypes of adenosine receptors. There has been evidence showing that the A_1 and A_{2A} adenosine receptors could form functional heteromers and directly interact with dopamine receptors (Ferre 2008; Ferre et al. 2008; Ferre et al. 1992; Fisone et al. 2004; Powell et al. 2001). Recent research has demonstrated that dopaminergic neurotransmission in the mesocorticolimbic rewarding circuit plays an important role in the mediation of the conditioned motivational effect of food cues (Ball et al. 2011; Floresco et al. 2008; Guy et al. 2011). Adenosine receptors exert a negative modulatory role in the dopaminergic rewarding system and caffeine antagonism of the adenosine receptors resulted in an enhanced dopaminergic activity (Cardinal 2006; Cauli and Morelli 2005; Daly et al. 1981; Daly and Fredholm 1998). Taken together, it is proposed that the caffeine-facilitated dopaminergic activities may underlie the enhanced responding-reinstating effect of food cue by pre-session administration of caffeine. In terms of the relative role of adenosine receptor subtypes, several studies have demonstrated that the antagonistic action of caffeine on adenosine A_{2A} receptors relative to A_1 subtype may play a main role in mediating the stimulant properties of caffeine (El Yacoubi et al. 2000a; El Yacoubi et al. 2000b; Halldner et al. 2004; Svenningsson et al. 1997). The mechanisms involving interactions between adenosine and dopamine receptors responsible for the enhancing effect of caffeine on cue-induced food-seeking behavior deserves future experimental investigation.

ACKNOWLEDGMENTS

This work was supported by National Institutes of Health grant DA017288 from the National Institute on Drug Abuse and funds from the Department of Psychiatry and Human Behavior, University of Mississippi Medical Center. The author would like to thank Ms./Mr. Courtney Jernigan, Lisa Biswas, Laura Beloate, Ramachandram Avusula, Treniea Tolliver, and Trisha Patel for their excellent technical assistance.

REFERENCES

Alvarez-Jaimes L, Polis I, Parsons LH (2008) Attenuation of cue-induced heroin-seeking behavior by cannabinoid CB1 antagonist infusions into the nucleus accumbens core and prefrontal cortex, but not basolateral amygdala. *Neuropsychopharmacology* 33: 2483-93.

Antoniou K, Kafetzopoulos E, Papadopoulou-Daifoti Z, Hyphantis T, Marselos M (1998) D-amphetamine, cocaine and caffeine: a comparative study of acute effects on locomotor activity and behavioural patterns in rats. *Neurosci. Biobehav. Rev.* 23: 189-96.

Aranda M, Morlock G (2006) Simultaneous determination of riboflavin, pyridoxine, nicotinamide, caffeine and taurine in energy drinks by planar chromatography-multiple detection with confirmation by electrospray ionization mass spectrometry. *J. Chromatogr. A* 1131: 253-60.

Ball KT, Combs TA, Beyer DN (2011) Opposing roles for dopamine D(1)- and D(2)-like receptors in discrete cue-induced reinstatement of food seeking. *Behav. Brain Res.* 222:390-3.

Bedingfield JB, King DA, Holloway FA (1998) Cocaine and caffeine: conditioned place preference, locomotor activity, and additivity. *Pharmacol. Biochem. Behav.* 61: 291-6.

Boutrel B, Koob GF (2004) What keeps us awake: the neuropharmacology of stimulants and wakefulness-promoting medications. *Sleep* 27: 1181-94.

Brunye TT, Mahoney CR, Lieberman HR, Giles GE, Taylor HA (2010) Acute caffeine consumption enhances the executive control of visual attention in habitual consumers. *Brain Cogn.* 74: 186-92.

Burbassi S, Cervo L (2008) Stimulation of serotonin2C receptors influences cocaine-seeking behavior in response to drug-associated stimuli in rats. *Psychopharmacology* (Berl) 196: 15-27.

Caballero M, Nunez F, Ahern S, Cuffi ML, Carbonell L, Sanchez S, Fernandez-Duenas V, Ciruela F (2011) Caffeine improves attention deficit in neonatal 6-OHDA lesioned rats, an animal model of attention deficit hyperactivity disorder (ADHD). *Neurosci. Lett.* 494: 44-8.

Cardinal RN (2006) Neural systems implicated in delayed and probabilistic reinforcement. *Neural Netw.* 19: 1277-301.

Carney JM (1982) Effects of caffeine, theophylline and theobromine on scheduled controlled responding in rats. *Br. J. Pharmacol.* 75: 451-4.

Cauli O, Morelli M (2005) Caffeine and the dopaminergic system. *Behav. Pharmacol.* 16: 63-77.

Ciccocioppo R, Sanna PP, Weiss F (2001) Cocaine-predictive stimulus induces drug-seeking behavior and neural activation in limbic brain regions after multiple months of abstinence: reversal by D(1) antagonists. *Proc. Natl. Acad. Sci. U. S. A.* 98: 1976-81.

Cohen C, Welzl H, Battig K (1991) Effects of nicotine, caffeine, and their combination on locomotor activity in rats. *Pharmacol. Biochem. Behav.* 40: 121-3.

Comer SD, Haney M, Foltin RW, Fischman MW (1997) Effects of caffeine withdrawal on humans living in a residential laboratory. *Exp. Clin. Psychopharmacol.* 5: 399-403.

Daly JW, Burns RE, Snyder SH (1981) Adenosine receptors in the central nervous system: Relationship. *Life Sci.* 28: 2083-97.

Daly JW, Fredholm BB (1998) Caffeine--an atypical drug of dependence. *Drug Alcohol. Depend.* 51: 199-206.

Depoortere RY, Li DH, Lane JD, Emmett-Oglesby MW (1993) Parameters of self-administration of cocaine in rats under a progressive-ratio schedule. *Pharmacol. Biochem. Behav.* 45: 539-48.

Ferre S (2008) An update on the mechanisms of the psychostimulant effects of caffeine. *J. Neurochem.* 105: 1067-79.

Ferre S, Ciruela F, Borycz J, Solinas M, Quarta D, Antoniou K, Quiroz C, Justinova Z, Lluis C, Franco R, Goldberg SR (2008) Adenosine A1-A2A receptor heteromers: new targets for caffeine in the brain. *Front Biosci.* 13: 2391-9.

Ferre S, Fuxe K, von Euler G, Johansson B, Fredholm BB (1992) Adenosine-dopamine interactions in the brain. *Neuroscience* 51: 501-12.

Fisone G, Borgkvist A, Usiello A (2004) Caffeine as a psychomotor stimulant: mechanism of action. *Cell Mol. Life Sci.* 61: 857-72.

Floresco SB, McLaughlin RJ, Haluk DM (2008) Opposing roles for the nucleus accumbens core and shell in cue-induced reinstatement of food-seeking behavior. *Neuroscience* 154: 877-84.

Frary CD, Johnson RK, Wang MQ (2005) Food sources and intakes of caffeine in the diets of persons in the United States. *J. Am. Diet Assoc.* 105: 110-3.

Fredholm BB, Battig K, Holmen J, Nehlig A, Zvartau EE (1999) Actions of caffeine in the brain with special reference to factors that contribute to its widespread use. *Pharmacol. Rev.* 51: 83-133.

Garrett BE, Holtzman SG (1994) D1 and D2 dopamine receptor antagonists block caffeine-induced stimulation of locomotor activity in rats. *Pharmacol. Biochem. Behav.* 47: 89-94.

Glade MJ (2010) Caffeine-Not just a stimulant. Nutrition 26: 932-8.

Gracy KN, Dankiewicz LA, Weiss F, Koob GF (2000) Heroin-specific stimuli reinstate operant heroin-seeking behavior in rats after prolonged extinction. *Pharmacol. Biochem. Behav.* 65: 489-94.

Green TA, Schenk S (2002) Dopaminergic mechanism for caffeine-produced cocaine seeking in rats. *Neuropsychopharmacology* 26: 422-30.

Guy EG, Choi E, Pratt WE (2011) Nucleus accumbens dopamine and mu-opioid receptors modulate the reinstatement of food-seeking behavior by food-associated cues. *Behav. Brain Res.* 219: 265-72.

Halldner L, Aden U, Dahlberg V, Johansson B, Ledent C, Fredholm BB (2004) The adenosine A1 receptor contributes to the stimulatory, but not the inhibitory effect of caffeine on locomotion: a study in mice lacking adenosine A1 and/or A2A receptors. *Neuropharmacology* 46: 1008-17.

Jaszyna M, Gasior M, Shoaib M, Yasar S, Goldberg SR (1998) Behavioral effects of nicotine, amphetamine and cocaine under a fixed-interval schedule of food reinforcement in rats chronically exposed to caffeine. *Psychopharmacology* (Berl) 140: 257-71.

Jessen A, Buemann B, Toubro S, Skovgaard IM, Astrup A (2005) The appetite-suppressant effect of nicotine is enhanced by caffeine. *Diabetes Obes. Metab.* 7: 327-33.

Katner SN, Magalong JG, Weiss F (1999) Reinstatement of alcohol-seeking behavior by drug-associated discriminative stimuli after prolonged extinction in the rat. *Neuropsychopharmacology* 20: 471-9.

Kuzmin A, Johansson B, Zvartau EE, Fredholm BB (1999) Caffeine, acting on adenosine A(1) receptors, prevents the extinction of cocaine-seeking behavior in mice. *J. Pharmacol. Exp. Ther.* 290: 535-42.

Liu X, Jernigan C (2012) Effects of caffeine on persistence and reinstatement of nicotine-seeking behavior in rats: interaction with nicotine-associated cues. *Psychopharmacology* (Berl) 220: 541-50.

Marin MT, Zancheta R, Paro AH, Possi AP, Cruz FC, Planeta CS (2011) Comparison of caffeine-induced locomotor activity between adolescent and adult rats. *Eur. J. Pharmacol.* 660: 363-7.

Packaged-Facts (2007) Energy drinks in the US, Rockville, MD.

Perkins KA, Fonte C, Stolinski A, Blakesley-Ball R, Wilson AS (2005) The influence of caffeine on nicotine's discriminative stimulus, subjective, and reinforcing effects. *Exp. Clin. Psychopharmacol.* 13: 275-81.

Pettenuzzo LF, Noschang C, von Pozzer Toigo E, Fachin A, Vendite D, Dalmaz C (2008) Effects of chronic administration of caffeine and stress on feeding behavior of rats. *Physiol. Behav.* 95: 295-301.

Powell KR, Iuvone PM, Holtzman SG (2001) The role of dopamine in the locomotor stimulant effects and tolerance to these effects of caffeine. *Pharmacol. Biochem. Behav.* 69: 59-70.

Racotta IS, Leblanc J, Richard D (1994) The effect of caffeine on food intake in rats: involvement of corticotropin-releasing factor and the sympatho-adrenal system. *Pharmacol. Biochem. Behav.* 48: 887-92.

Rezvani AH, Sexton HG, Johnson J, Wells C, Gordon K, Levin ED (2013) Effects of caffeine on alcohol consumption and nicotine self-administration in rats. *Alcohol. Clin. Exp. Res.* 37: 1609-17.

Schenk S, Partridge B (1999) Cocaine-seeking produced by experimenter-administered drug injections: dose-effect relationships in rats. *Psychopharmacology* (Berl) 147: 285-90.

Schenk S, Worley CM, McNamara C, Valadez A (1996) Acute and repeated exposure to caffeine: effects on reinstatement of extinguished cocaine-taking behavior in rats. *Psychopharmacology* (Berl) 126: 17-23.

Tremblay A, Masson E, Leduc S, Houde A, Despres JP (1988) Caffeine reduces spontaneous energy intake in men but not in women. *Nutrition Research* 8: 553-8.

Uslaner JM, Drott JT, Sharik SS, Theberge CR, Sur C, Zeng Z, Williams DL, Hutson PH (2010) Inhibition of glycine transporter 1 attenuates nicotine- but not food-induced cue-potentiated reinstatement for a response previously paired with sucrose. *Behav. Brain Res.* 207: 37-43.

Wing VC, Shoaib M (2008) Contextual stimuli modulate extinction and reinstatement in rodents self-administering intravenous nicotine. *Psychopharmacology* (Berl) 200: 357-65.

Wood S, Sage JR, Shuman T, Anagnostaras SG (2014) Psychostimulants and cognition: a continuum of behavioral and cognitive activation. *Pharmacol. Rev.* 66: 193-221.

Worley CM, Valadez A, Schenk S (1994) Reinstatement of extinguished cocaine-taking behavior by cocaine and caffeine. *Pharmacol. Biochem. Behav.* 48: 217-21.

In: Caffeine
Editor: Aimée S. Tolley

ISBN: 978-1-63117-777-4
© 2014 Nova Science Publishers, Inc.

Chapter 3

CAFFEINE: FORMS OF CONSUMPTION, TOXICITY, THERAPEUTIC EFFECTS AND THEIR USE IN MEDICINE

ABSTRACT

Caffeinated drinks (coffee and others) and tea are the most consumed, socially-acceptable stimulants in the world. In their natural forms, coffee and tea contain several chemical components that may confer both beneficial and adverse health effects,

Caffeine, a methylxanthine, is closely related to theophylline. Caffeine is rapidly and completely absorbed from the gastrointestinal tract. The volume of distribution in adults is approximately 0.5 L/kg. Caffeine is primarily metabolized by the cytochrome P450 (CYP) oxidase system in the liver. The plasma half-life of caffeine varies considerably from person to person, with an average half-life of 5-8 hours in healthy, nonsmoking adults. Caffeine clearance is accelerated in smokers; clearance is slowed in pregnancy, in liver disease, and in the presence of some CYP inhibitors.

There is insufficient evidence for promoting or discouraging coffee consumption in the daily diet. Caffeine consumption has multiple systemic effects, involving the neuropsychiatric, cardiovascular, endocrine-metabolic, genitourinary and gastrointestinal systems. The impact on health may be modified by genetic factors, age, sex, medications, and other environmental exposures.

It is used for treating of idiopathic apnea of prematurity, acute respiratory depression, restore mental alertness o wakefulness when experiencing fatigue, and less frequently for treating spinal puncture headache, diuretic, augmentation of seizure induction during electroconvulsive therapy, and acute migraine (combined with indomethacyn and prochlorperazine).

This review will focus on the consumption of caffeine, its role on neurologic performance, sport and some specific disease processes, explaining side effects, toxicity, caffeine dependence, withdrawal and tolerance.

Dr. S. Castaño

INTRODUCTION

Dr. A. Martín, RN. E. Montial and Dr. M. Iturbe

History of Caffeine in Nature and Products

Caffeine is a natural substance that is present in over 60 plant species. Alternative names include theine, guaranine and mateine. It is consumed by humans in the form of beverages such as coffee, tea, chocolate and soft drinks. Coffee was first discovered in Arabia during the 9th century, and was originally cultivated in Ethiopia. Tea was first drunk in China and cacao was discovered in South America. During the 15th century, coffee became popular all over the world. The most common species of coffee are *Coffea arabica* (Arabica coffee) and *Coffea canephora* (Robusta coffee), which respectively account for 80-90% and 10-20% of worldwide production. Coffee is the product which contains the highest and most variable quantity of caffeine in the human diet (between 0.8-1.8%). The amount of caffeine present in coffee depends on the genetic make-up of the coffee beans themselves, as well as the time and method of preparation, and generally oscillates between 30 and 175 mg per 150 ml. Decaffeinated coffee contains between 2 and 8 mg per 150 ml [1].

The natural product that contains the second highest amount of caffeine is tea, a beverage made from the dried leaves of the *Camellia* or *Thea sinensis, bohea* or *viridis* bush. There are 4 types of tea: green, red, black and white, depending on the processing methods used. These processing methods also affect the concentration of caffeine in the final beverage, which can vary between 20 and 73 mg/100 ml [1].

Cacao contains the third highest concentration of caffeine, and is obtained from the seeds of the *Theobroma cacao* (cacao tree). The proportion of caffeine in this product is 0.4%. The caffeine content of chocolate is between 5 and 20 mg/100 g. Dark, bitter or semi-sweet chocolate contains much more caffeine than milk chocolate [1].

Other plants such as guarana (Paullina cupana), yerba mate (Ilex paraguariensis), kola nuts (Cola nitida) and yoco also contain a 2-4% proportion of caffeine [1].

A number of other beverages also exist with variable caffeine content. These include soft drinks and energy drinks, the latter of which contain a higher percentage of caffeine [1].

Some medical drugs also contain caffeine in combination with other active ingredients, with content oscillating between 15 and 200 mg [1].

In general, the main source of caffeine in the average adult diet is coffee. In children under the age of 18, the average intake of caffeine is 1 mg/kg/day, and the main sources are soft drinks and chocolate. The Food and Drug Administration (FDA) has set the limit for the amount of caffeine permitted in carbonated soft drinks at 0.2 mg/ml and obliges producers to state the quantity of caffeine contained in the beverage on its label whenever it is added intentionally. In 2003, a European regulation was passed which extends Directive 2002/67/EC and states that beverages containing more than 150 mg/L of caffeine must indicate this fact clearly on the label. Some countries have their own laws regarding the commercial control and consumption of energy drinks [1].

Caffeine is a substance with both beneficial and harmful systematic effects. While it can be used for therapeutic purposes, its adverse effects and interactions should always be borne in mind both during use and in the treatment of overdoses. This chapter provides a detailed description of the pharmacological properties of caffeine and its clinical use, as well as the treatment indicated for possible complications related to this substance.

Biochemical Properties [2]

Caffeine (methylated xanthine 1,3,7-trimethylxantine) is a highly soluble compound that readily crosses cell membranes throughout the body. It is rapidly absorbed in the stomach and small intestine and can be detected in human tissues 30 to 45 minutes after ingestion, with peak blood concentration reached within two hours. The biochemical formula for caffeine is 1,3,7-trimethylxanthine (Figure 1).

Caffeine is rapidly and almost completely absorbed by the gastrointestinal tract and quickly diffuses into all body tissues. Its half-life ranges from 2.5 to 10 hours, and after an oral intake, a rapid plasma peak is observed after between 45 minutes and 2 hours. The wide spectrum of serum half-life concentration is determined by the relevant inter-individual variability, which in turn is related to several genetic and environmental factors.

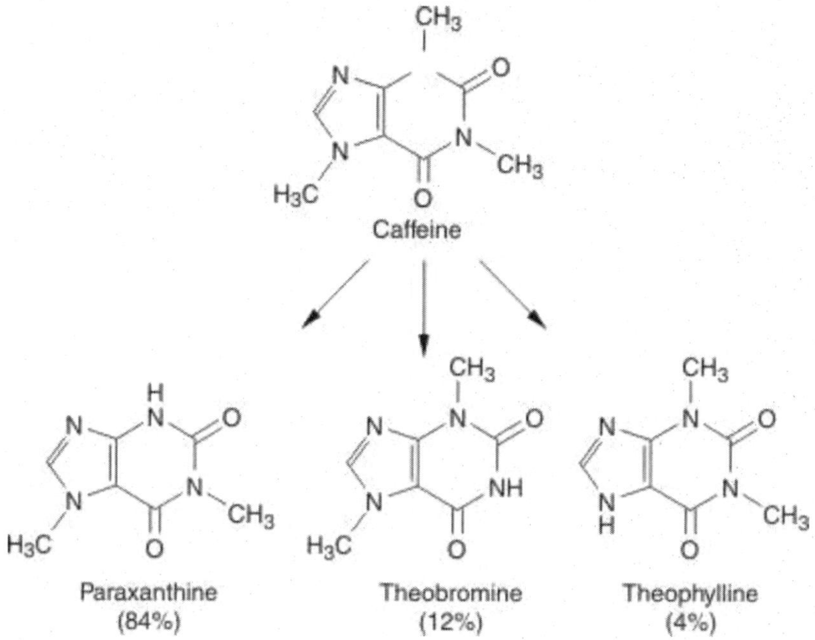

Figure 1. Biochemical structure and metabolism of caffeine [6].

Caffeine is metabolised by liver microsomes (P450 microsomes) that can be induced by the caffeine itself or other xenobiotics inhaled or ingested by the subject, such as smoke, medicines or alcohol. Caffeine is metabolised to approximately 95% in more than 25 derived molecules (the principal ones being 3,7-theobromine, 1,3-theophylline and 1,7-paraxanthine). It has a bioavailability of 100%. It binds to plasma proteins, mainly albumin, at a percentage of between 10% and 35% and its volume of distribution is 0.6 to 0.7 L/kg. It quickly passes through the cell membranes, including the placental blood-brain membrane. It is metabolised in the liver through demethylation by CYP1A2. 25 metabolites have been described. Plasma concentrations vary from one individual to another, due to variations in each person's metabolism. 95% of caffeine is metabolised through demethylation by the CYP1A2 subfamily of the cytochrome P450 isoenzyme. To a lesser extent, it is also metabolised by other enzymes such as CYP2E1 and CYP3A3. Its elimination is non-linear at high doses due to enzymatic saturation, and occurs after the caffeine metabolism. Only 1-2% is eliminated unaltered in urine. The rest is eliminated in urine in the form of more polar metabolites, such as paraxantine and theophylline, the biological activity of which is similar to that of caffeine. Caffeine is secreted in breast milk, saliva, bile and semen. Its elimination half-life is 3-5 hours. In newborns and babies up to the age of 3-6 months, both its metabolism and renal clearance are much lower, with a half-life of up to 100 hours. In smokers and individuals who do not usually drink coffee, its half-life is twice as long, which explains the greater prevalence of overdoses in this population [3-5].

Mechanism of Action

Like other methylxanthines, caffeine has multiple pharmacological effects, including adenosine receptor antagonism, presynaptic $\alpha 1$ receptor antagonism and phosphodiesterase inhibition, which results in increased catecholamine release, and A-adrenergic receptor stimulation.

Caffeine stimulates the central nervous system and, in general, increases cyclic AMP. Caffeine acts through different molecular pathways, resulting in a wide range of biological effects [2,4].

a) Adenosine Receptors

The action and effect of adenosine on the body's different physiological systems are generally the opposite of the action and effect of caffeine. Caffeine is a methylxanthine which, being similar to purine, binds to the A1 and A2a adenosine receptors. The majority of caffeine's pharmacological effects seem to depend on the antagonistic action of adenosine in cell surface receptors. At the plasma concentrations found following mean caffeine intake in an adult diet, caffeine is the non-selective antagonist of the A1 and A2a adenosine receptors. Caffeine acts by inhibiting the A1, A2a and A2b adenosine receptors and has a low affinity for A3 receptors [1,4].

b) Phosphodiesterases

Caffeine is a weak competitive inhibitor of phosphodiesterase, increasing the effect and duration of intracellular cAMP. The result is a strengthening of the effects of catecholamines [4].

c) Calcium Channels

Caffeine activates the ryanodine-sensitive calcium channels found in the endoplasmic and sarcoplasmic reticula, triggering the release of intracellular calcium and affecting calcium homeostasis. Doses much higher than the therapeutic concentration of caffeine are required to trigger these effects, which become particularly acute in the event of overdose [4].

d) GABAa Receptors

Caffeine acts as an antagonist in the binding sites of benzodiazepine, which blocks the GABAa receptors. Nevertheless, the concentration of caffeine required to produce this effect is much greater than that commonly reached as part of a normal adult diet [4].

e) Others

Other areas in which caffeine acts include various ion channels, with the release of neurotransmitters, and a number of different enzymes. In general, this effect is inhibitory in nature. Effects on calcium entry and potassium and calcium channels have also been described. Caffeine also seems to increase the sensitivity of Mg-ATPase to the stimulating effects of calcium in the cardiac myofibrils [4].

Nutritional Value

Neither caffeine nor any of its metabolites described above provide our organism with macronutrients, and since they do not form part of the Krebs Cycle, neither can they be considered a source of energy (Kcal). Caffeine and its derivatives competitively and non-selectively inhibit phosphodiesterase [7], thus increasing intracellular cAMP, and bind to the non-selective adenosine receptor antagonist [8].

Thus, the acute administration of caffeine results in a 5%-25% increase in the basal metabolic rate, and therefore the total energy expenditure (TEE). These changes in the energy metabolism have been associated with significant increases in serum concentrations of fatty acids, glycerol and lactate, due to the lipolytic effect produced by phosphodiesterase inhibition [7], the release of catecholamines and adenosine receptor antagonism.

2. CAFFEINE CONSUMPTION

Dr. M. Iturbe, Dr. A. Martín and Dr. A. Quintano

Forms of Consumption / Amount Present in Medical Drugs and Common Food Stuffs

Caffeine is consumed by humans mainly in the form of infusions extracted from the fruit of the coffee plant and the leaves of the tea bush, as well as in beverages and food stuffs which contain products derived from kola nuts.

Caffeine can access our organism either orally or rectally, as well as intramuscularly and intravenously in the case of pharmacological administration.

There are more than 50 plants which contain this active ingredient in their leaves, seeds or fruit. The following are the most important [5,9].

Coffee (Coffea arabica). One of the primary sources of caffeine throughout the world is the coffee bean (the seed of the coffee plant), which is used to make the beverage known as coffee. The caffeine content of coffee varies widely depending on the type of coffee bean in question and the preparation method used (even beans from the same bush may have different caffeine concentrations) [5].

Yoco or huarmiyoco (Paullina yoco) contains the second highest concentration of caffeine. Caffeine is found in the bark of the yoco tree in proportions almost as high as in coffee. The beverage is prepared by scraping off the bark and then squeezing it in order to extract its sap, which is then mixed with water [5].

Kola nuts (Cola nitida Vent.) come originally from Africa. Caffeine is present in the dried, shelled seeds of various species of the Cola genus, particularly Cola nitida and Cola acuminata. Cola acuminata is an African tree with caffeine-containing seeds or nuts. The caffeine concentration of kola nuts is similar to that of coffee and yoco, although it is released more slowly, thus producing a milder but longer-lasting effect [5].

Guarana (Paullinia cupana HBK) is a tropical climbing plant native to South America. Caffeine is contained in its seeds, which are usually shelled before being roasted and ground into a powder.

Table 1. Caffeinated content in coffee

Volume/weight	Mean Caffeine Range (mg)
Coffee	
Roasted coffee 100 mL	41-83 (60)
Instant coffee 100mL	27-72 (50)
Decaffeinated roasted coffee 100 mL	0.4-7.2 (4)
Decaffeinated instant coffee 100mL	1-5 (3)
Dunkin' Donuts Coffee with Turbo Shot *(large, 20 fl. oz.)*	436
Starbucks Coffee *(venti, 20 fl. oz.)*	415
Panera Frozen Mocha *(16.5 fl. oz.)*	267
Starbucks Caffè Americano (large, 16 fl. oz.)	225
Dunkin' Donuts Coffee (medium, 14 fl. oz.)	178
Starbucks Iced Coffee (large, 16 fl. oz.)	165
Starbucks Espresso (doppio, 2 fl. oz.)	150
Keurig Coffee K-Cup, all varieties (1 cup, makes 8 fl. oz.)	75-150
Folgers Classic Roast Instant Coffee (2 tsp., makes 12 fl. oz.)	148
Starbucks Doubleshot Energy Coffee, can (15 fl. oz.)	146
Starbucks Mocha Frappuccino (venti, 24 fl. oz.)	140
Starbucks VIA House Blend Instant Coffee (1 packet, makes 8 fl. oz.)	135
McDonald's Coffee (large, 16 fl. oz.)	133
International Delight Iced Coffee (8 fl. oz.)	76
Maxwell House Lite Ground Coffee (2 Tbs., makes 12 fl. oz.)	50-70
Dunkin' Donuts, Panera, or Starbucks Decaf Coffee (16 fl. oz.)	15-25

Huito or jagua (Genipa americana). A tree native to America whose seeds have a high caffeine content [5].

Yerba mate or Paraguayan tea (Ilex paraguariensis). The leaves of this bush are a rich source of caffeine. They are dried and roasted and then steeped in hot water to make the beverage also known as mate [5].

Cacao (Theobroma cacao). The seeds of the cacao tree contain about half the amount of caffeine as the plants listed above. This food staff contains a series of other components, including phenylethylamine, which belongs to the amphetamine family, although it is also rich in alkaloids such as caffeine and theobromine [5].

Tea (Camellia sinensis Kuntze). Caffeine is found in the leaves and throughout the whole plant in general. Tea is a very common source of caffeine. Although tea itself contains more caffeine than coffee, a typical portion of this beverage contains much less, since it is normally prepared as a much more diluted infusion [5].

Other plants with contain much smaller quantities of caffeine in their flowers include:

- The lemon tree (Citrus limon).
- The grapefruit tree (Citrus paradisi).
- The orange tree (Citrus sinensis).

As mentioned earlier, caffeine is found in numerous different commercial products and medicines (Tables 1-7 [1,2,5,10-14]). In addition to the natural caffeine obtained as the result of the industrial decaffeination process, caffeine can also be obtained by theobromine methylation as well as through total chemical synthesis, using dimethylcarbamide and malonic acid.

Table 2. Caffeine content in tea

Volume/weight	Mean Caffeine Range (mg)
Tea	
Black tea 100mL	10-46 (25)
Green tea 100mL	8-17 (12)
White tea 100mL	2-11 (6)
Red tea 100 mL	5-30 (18)
Iced tea 100mL	4-21 (12)
Starbucks Tazo Awake—Brewed Tea or Tea Latte (large, 16 fl. oz.)	135
Starbucks Tazo Chai Tea Latte (large, 16 fl. oz.)	95
Black tea, brewed for 3 minutes (8 fl. oz.)	30-80
Snapple Lemon Tea (16 fl. oz.)	62
Lipton Pure Leaf Iced Tea (18.5 fl. oz.)	60
Lipton 100% Natural Lemon Iced Tea, bottle (20 fl. oz.)	35
Arizona Iced Tea, black, all varieties (16 fl. oz.)	30
Nestea Unsweetened Iced Tea Mix (2 tsp., makes 8 fl. oz.)	20-30
Black tea 100mL	10-46 (25)
Green tea 100mL	8-17 (12)
White tea 100mL	2-11 (6)
Red tea 100 mL	5-30 (18)
Iced tea 100mL	4-21 (12)
Herbal tea, brewed (8 fl. oz.)	0

Table 3. Caffeine content in chocolate candy and chocolate drinks

Volume/weight	Mean Caffeine Range (mg)
Chocolate Candy & Chocolate Drinks	
Cacao bean 100g	0.1-0.5 (0.2)
Powdered cacao 10g	10-16 (12)
Dark chocolate 100g	17-118 (68)
White chocolate 100g	0
Bitter chocolate 100g	16-34 (24)
Milk chocolate 100g	1-38 (20)
Hot chocolate drink 100ml	1-49 (34)
Chocolate milk 100ml	1-7 (3)

Table 4. Caffeine content in energy drinks

Volume/weight	Mean Caffeine Range (mg)
Energy Drinks (16 fl. oz. unless noted)	
RedLine Power Rush (2.5 fl. oz.)	350
Ammo (1 fl. oz.)	171
Powershot (1 fl. oz.)	100
Fuel Cell (2 fl. oz.)	180
Wired X505 (24 fl. oz.)	505
Fixx (20 fl. oz.)	500
BooKoo Energy (24 fl. oz.)	360
Wired X344 (16 fl. oz.)	344
SPIKE Shooter (8.4 fl. oz.)	300
Viso Energy Vigor (20fl. oz.)	300
Cocaine Energy Drink (8.4 fl. oz.)	280
Jolt Cola (23.5 fl. oz.)	280
NOS (16 fl. oz.)	250
Redline RTD (8 fl. oz.)	250
Blow (Energy Drink Mix)(8 fl. oz.)	240
5-hour Energy (1.9 fl. oz.)	208
Full Throttle	200
No Fear 16	174
Monster Energy	160
Rockstar	160
AMP Energy Boost Original	142
TaB Energy 10.5	95
Red Bull (8.4 fl. oz.)	80
V8 V-Fusion+Energy (8 fl. oz.)	80
SoBe Adrenaline Rush (8.3 fl. oz.)	79
Ocean Spray Cran-Energy (8 fl. oz.)	55
Starbucks Refreshers (12 fl. oz.)	50
Energy drinks 330ml	9-12(10)
Drinks containing guarana 330 mL	0.1-12 (8)
Guarana paste 100g	2.5-5 (4)
Mate 100mL	0.2 - 2 (1.5)

Caffeine 45

Table 5. Caffeine content in soft drinks

Volume/weight	Mean Caffeine Range (mg)
Soft Drinks (12 fl. oz.)	
Cola 330mL	3-7 (4)
Decaffeinated cola 330mL	0
Diet cola	2-7 (4)
Decaffeinated diet cola	0
Pepsi MAX	69
Mountain Dew—Diet or regular	54
Diet Coke	47
Pepsi	38
Coca-Cola, Coke Zero or Diet Pepsi	35
Barq's Root Beer, regular	23
7-Up, Fanta, Fresca, ginger ale or Sprite	0

Table 6. Caffeine content in ice cream and yogurt

Volume/weight	Mean Caffeine Range (mg)
Ice Cream & Yogurt (4 oz. unless noted)	
Cold Stone Creamery Mocha Ice Cream (Gotta Have It, 12 oz.)	52
Starbucks Coffee Ice Cream	45
TCBY Coffee Frozen Yogurt (large, 13.4 fl. oz.)	42
Dannon All Natural Coffee Low fat Yogurt (6 oz.)	30
Häagen-Dazs Coffee Ice Cream	29
Baskin Robbins Jamoca Ice Cream	20
Dreyer's or Edy's Grand Ice Cream—Coffee or Espresso Chip	17
Breyers Coffee Ice Cream	11
Dreyer's, Edy's, or Häagen-Dazs Chocolate Ice Cream	<1
Non-prescription medicines – 1 dose	36-200 (102)

Table 7. Caffeine content in Medicines

Medicines	Caffeine (mg)
EXCEDRIN tab.	65
ASPIRINA PLUS	50
CAFIASPIRINA	50
MEJORAL CAFEÍNA	30
CAFEÍNA CITRATO vial.	20/mL
PEYONA vial.	20/mL
CAFERGOT	100
BIODRAMINA CAFEÍNA tab.	50
OKALDOL CAFEÍNA chewable tab.	30
CALMAGRIP FORTE powder for oral sol.	25
COFIGRIP powder	25
COLFORT powder for oral sol.	25
DOLVIRAN tab.	50
GRIPESTOP powder for oral sol.	25
ILVICO tab.	30
LAFOR powder	25
NORVOGRIP powder	25
OPTALIDON lozenge	25
OPTALIDON sup.	75
SALDEVA FORTE tab.	50
TONOPAN film-coated tab.	40
CAFINITRINA sublingual tab.	25
CALMANTE DENTAL BROTA sachet	60/120
FRENADOL COMPLEX granules for oral sol.	20
ACTRON COMPUESTO effervescent tab.	40
ANALGILASA film-coated tab.	30
CALMAGRIP tab.	25
CALMANTE VITAMINADO PEREZ GIMENEZ tab.	50
CINFAMAR CAFEÍNA film-coated tab.	50
DESENFRIOL-C GRANULADO powder sachet	32.4
DURVITAN show-release cap.	300
DYNAMÍN film-coated tab.	30
EXCEDITE film-coated tab.	65
HEMICRANEAL tab.	300
LAFOR powder for oral sol.	25
NEOCIBALENA tab.	50
CAFNEA oral	25
CAFNEA vial	20/mL

3. Direct Effects of Caffeine

Dr. B. Fernández-Miret, Dr. M. Prieto and Dr. H. Barrasa

Caffeine, like the rest of methylxanthines, produces a number of effects in different organs and systems. It differs from theophylline by the addition of a single methyl group. Methylxanthines are hypothesized to have multiple mechanisms of action, including phosphodiesterase (PDE) inhibition, adenosine receptor antagonism, and release of catecholamines. At therapeutic doses, this results in bronchodilation, increased gastric acid secretion, headache, nausea, vomiting, diuresis, tachycardia, and central nervous system (CNS) excitation (see Table 8) [12]. The most characteristic effect is the psycho-stimulant effect on the CNS, but caffeine also affects other, but not less important, systems.

Table 8. Pharmacology of methylxantines [12]

Clinical effect	Mechanism
Bronchodilation	PDE-4 inhibition, A_1 antagonism
Increased gastric secretions	PDE-4 inhibition
Headache, vomiting	PDE-4 inhibition, catecholamine release
Diuresis	A_1 antagonism
Tachycardia	PDE-3 inhibition, A_1 antagonism, catecholamine release
Hypotension	B_2 adrenergic agonism
CNS excitation	A_1 antagonism, catecholamine release

A: adenosine; CNS: central nervous system; PDE: phosphodiesterase.

Central Nervous System

Cognitive/stimulating effect: Caffeine produces shaped dose-dependent generalized activation of CNS, probably by increasing the release of norepinephrine [15]. Increases alertness, reduces tiredness and fatigue, increases the ability to maintain an intellectual effort and maintains wakefulness despite sleep deprivation. Moreover, by inhibiting the A2 receptor, caffeine has a reinforcing action by the release of dopamine in the brain reward circuitry (mesolimbic system and nucleus accumbens). This action could be explained by an increased phosphorylation of DARPP-32 (phosphoprotein regulating dopamine and cAMP).

In rested individuals, moderate and low doses of caffeine, about 30 to 300 mg, improve alertness and reaction time [16]. In people with lack of sleep, the positive effects of caffeine are generalized to a wide variety of functions, including learning, decission making, increasing the ability of concentration [17]. This is probably the main reason why so many humans regularly consume caffeine. A systematic review of 13 randomized trials of people with jet lag or shift work disorder found that caffeine significantly improves the formation of concepts, reasoning, memory, orientation, attention and perception, compared with placebo [18]. Caffeine is also found to be better than placebo in preventing of errors and was equally effective compared with other active interventions such as the use of modafinil or bright light.

Effect on cerebral blood flow: Most studies have found that caffeine induces a global cerebral vasoconstriction with resultant decreased cerebral blood flow, although this effect may not occur in people over 65 years. According to recent research, no tolerance develops to these vasoconstrictor effects and cerebral blood flow shows an increase in the rebound after caffeine abstinence [19].

Analgesic effect: Caffeine has a dose-dependent analgesic effect enhanced by the serotonin inhibitors and an adjuvant effect on the analgesia. Caffeine has a long and known history as an adjuvant analgesic. In a review, the authors show preclinical studies of intrinsic antinociceptive action of caffeine. The antinociceptive dose varied between 25 and 100 mg.kg^{-1} [20]. The antinocicepcion seems to occur mainly by the blockade of adenosine A2a and A2b receptors. Other mechanisms not related with the blockade of adenosine, such as changes in the activity and the synthesis of cyclo-oxygenase enzymes in certain regions, are also involved in the adjuvant analgesic effect of caffeine.

Cardiovascular System

Caffeine administration causes an increase in blood pressure and has a positive chronotropic and inotropic effect by inhibition of the cardiac adenosine receptors, resulting in an increase in heart rate. However, they are not used as primary agents in the treatment of heart failure, since their stimulatory effect on the nervous system and potential adverse effects on cardiac rhythm outweigh any potential benefits of increased inotropy [21].

There is a widespread belief that caffeine, especially at high doses, is associated with palpitations and an increased number of arrhythmias, including atrial fibrillation and supraventricular and ventricular ectopy [22]. Electrophysiological studies have shown that caffeine has some effects that could promote arrhythmogenesis. However, there is no evidence that caffeine in doses typically consumed can provoke a spontaneous arrhythmia, or facilitate the induction of an arrhythmia in the electrophysiology laboratory [23].

Caffeine can acutely raise blood pressure to 10 mmHg in patients who are not regular users, which does not happen in regular coffee consumers [24]. With regard to coronary disease, the risk may be increased in persons who are slow metabolizers of caffeine and drink two or more cups of coffee a day [25].

Respiratory System

The use of methylxanthines such as treatment of respiratory disorders is widely held. Primarily stimulate the respiratory center and have bronchodilator effect. Theophylline is the most widely used clinically despite having a narrow therapeutic range and cause the most serious adverse effects [1]. The antitussive effect of theobromine is well known. Caffeine is also widely used to treat preterm infants apnea, with minimal adverse effects [26].

Respiratory stimulant effects of xanthine occur because of the antagonism of adenosine receptors on the respiratory center. Caffeine increases the sensitivity of the respiratory center to carbon dioxide. In cases of poisoning can occur respiratory alkalosis [27]. At the peripheral level, caffeine has an inhibitory effect on the respiration by the blockade of A2 adenosine receptors in the carotid body. Caffeine seems to improve lung function in asthmatics, probably because it increases the bronchodilator effect [28,29].

Renal System

Both caffeine and other methylxanthines cause vasodilation of the afferent arteriole of the renal glomerulus, which increases blood flow to the kidney and increases the glomerular filtration rate, related to the diuretic effect actions that produce these substances [30].

The available literature suggests that acute ingestion of caffeine in large doses (at least 250–300 mg, equivalent to the amount found in 2–3 cups of coffee or 5–8 cups of tea) results in a short-term stimulation of urine output in individuals who have been deprived of caffeine for a period of days or weeks. A profound tolerance to the diuretic and other effects of caffeine develops, however, and the actions are much diminished in individuals who regularly consume tea or coffee. Doses of caffeine equivalent to the amount normally found in standard servings of tea, coffee and carbonated soft drinks appear to have no diuretic action. Nowadays, there is no support for the suggestion that consumption of caffeine-containing beverages as part of a normal lifestyle leads to fluid loss in excess of the volume ingested or is associated with poor hydration status [31].

In addition to the diuretic effect, which happens by antagonizing A1 and A2a adenosine receptors [32], also presents natriuretic effect by which is used to treat edema associated with congestive heart failure.

Miscellaneus

Effects on musculoskeletal system:

Moderate consumption of caffeine causes increase of calcium in myocytes that increases striated muscle contractility and decreases muscle fatigue [33]. By antagonistic action of adenosine there is smooth muscle relaxation. On the other side it has been observed that high coffee intake may be associated with lower bone mineral density and increased fracture risk in women, particularly those with low calcium intake [34]. Moreover, in cases of poisoning may occur tremor, twitching, hypertonia, myoclonus an even rhabdomyolysis resulting from the increase of muscular activity and the direct citotoxicicidad by carboxyterminal calcium increase [35].

Gastrointestinal and methabolic effects:

Caffeine stimulates the contractions of the gallbladder, relaxes the smooth muscle of biliary tract, reduces cholesterol levels in bile and stimulates gastric acid secretion [36]. By the increase in gastric acid production can exacerbate or induce dyspepsia and increase gastroesophageal reflux. Have also been reported cases of emesis and nausea and even hyperemesis in patients with Mallory-Weiss Syndrome [37].

Caffeine causes a dose-dependent increase in total cholesterol, HDL, LDL and triglycerides, although it seems that this increase is not clinically relevant [38].

Effects of caffeine on reproductive outcomes in women:

Several basic research studies have assessed the effect of caffeine on trophoblast biology in vitro and suggested molecular mechanisms for deleterious caffeine effect on pregnancy outcomes. However the bulk of available evidence is low quality and suggests that mild to moderate caffeine intake is not associated with any adverse reproductive outcome. Despite of the physiological effects of caffeine exposure have not been studied extensively in human pregnancy, studies suggest fetal tolerance to caffeine exposure also appears to occur, although there have been described other fetal effects related to maternal caffeine consumption, like increased fetal heart rate variability, lower basal heart rate, and increased fetal breathing activity.

Potential adverse effects of caffeine consumption like uteroplacental vasoconstriction induced by the release of circulating catecholamines, or increases in maternal homocysteine, colesterol and changes in maternal reproductive hormone levels have not been proven [39].

Caffeine has been associated with alterations in estradiol and other hormones, which in turn may affect ovulation, the length of the follicular or luteal phase, or other menstrual characteristics. Caffeine has also been related to shorter menstrual cycle length and a lower risk of very long menstrual cycles. Soda, both with and without caffeine, has been associated with increased insulin resistance, metabolic syndrome, and weight gain, which in turn are related to polycystic ovary syndrome, a leading cause of ovulatory infertility [40].

Many researchers have studied about a possible relationship between caffeine and fecundability; most of prospective epidemiological studies have not found a statistically significant association between them. However, reproductive endocrinologists suggest that it may be prudent for women who are having difficulty conceiving to limit caffeine consumption to less than 200 to 300 mg per day, in addition to eliminating tobacco use and decreasing alcohol consumption. Caffeine consumption by the male partner does not appear to affect male fertility potential.

The relationship between spontaneous abortion adn caffeine exposure is not fairly proven. Many studies did not observe an association at any level of reported exposure. Studies that noted a link between caffeine intake and spontaneous abortion generally reported a dose-response relationship; an increased risk of spontaneous abortion generally was not observed until intake levels were ≥ 3 cups or ≥ 300 mg caffeine per day. This association were not found in the Danish national birth cohort with > 600 mg caffeine per day.

Although some of these epidemiologic studies reported an association between caffeine intake and certain congenital anomalies (e.g. anorectal atresia, congenital limb deffets, small intestinal atresia, craniosynostosis, anotia/microtia), the results should be interpreted with caution due to the methodological flaws of these studies (eg, lack of correction for multiple comparisons, poor ascertainment of caffeine intake, etiologic heterogeneity for some malformations, biased exposure data, biased ascertainment of congenital anomalies) or because the findings were inconsistent with basic teratological principles. Several narrative reviews and a systematic review concluded that caffeine is unlikely to cause congenital anomalies at doses consumed by humans (eg, fractional doses totaling <5 mg/kg body weight/day) [39].

A 2011 systematic review concluded it is unlikely that caffeine intake <300 mg/day has a significant adverse effect on fetal growth in non-smoking women.

A recently systematic review and a meta-analysis did not found a significant association between maternal caffeine intake anytime in pregnancy and preterm birth. Neither has been proven association between any source of exposure to caffeine from food in pregnancy and fetal mortality.

Several epidemiological studies of coffee consumption have showed that long-term coffee consumption is associated with reduced risk of diabetes. In a prospective cohort study, preconceptional moderate caffeine intake from coffee appeared to protect against development of gestational diabetes mellitus.

Although higher caffeine intake was associated with elevated systolic blood pressure in the first and third trimestersd caffeine consumption appeared to be protective against preeclampsia.

Caffeine is detectable in breast milk within 15 minutes of consumption and levels peak after about one hour. Adverse effects have not been reported in term infants whose mothers had moderate intake of up to five cups of coffee daily, but some case reports have described an increase in infant irritability, jitteriness, or sleep disturbance at this level of maternal caffeine consumption.

Caffeine Intake Recommendations

For women who are pregnant or trying to become pregnant, and breastfeeding mothers several associations suggest daily caffeine intake of no more than 200-300 mg/day [39].

4. CAFFEINE´S SIDE EFFECTS AND TOXICITY

Dr. S. Castaño, RN. E. Jiménez and Dr. F. J. Maynar

Acute Side Effects

Due to the large intersubject variability, the same dose of caffeine can cause adverse reactions in a person and have good tolerability in another one. Adults should limit their caffeine intake to 500 mg per day. Individuals who have heart problems, high blood pressure, or trouble sleeping or who are taking medications should be careful to limit the amount of caffeine they drink. Older and younger persons and may be more sensitive to the effects of caffeine [11]. The most common adverse effects are palpitation, tachycardia, gastric disturbances, tremor, nervousness and insomnia [1,4,41]. High doses can cause intense anxiety, fear and panic attacks. There have been reports of acute caffeine-induced psychosis in individuals without psychopathology or worsening of psychotic symptoms in schizophrenic. In addition, it can cause anaphylaxis [1,4].

Cardiovascular adverse effects: Caffeine does not induce or worsen the severity of ventricular arrhythmias and very high doses [42] predispose individuals to atrial flutter and atrial fibrillation, as well as atrioventricular nodal reentry tachycardia [12,43]. There are multiple recent studies of atrial fibrillation and supraventricular tachycardia associated with the use of caffeinated energy beverages [12,44]. Caffeine intake is also significantly correlated with elevated daytime systolic and diastolic blood pressure in African-American adolescents.

Hepatic adverse effects: jaundice, liver synthetic dysfunction and cholestatic hepatitis appear rarely [12].

Genitourinary adverse effects: caffeine promotes diuresis and increases detrusor pressure, which, together, might increase the likelihood of urgency-related involuntary urine loss [4]. Recent large epidemiological studies of women have revealed that caffeine is associated with prevalent urinary incontinence (UI) and incident urgency urinary incontinence [45-47]. However, a posterior prospective study did not confirmed this association, showing that long-term caffeine intake over 1 year was not associated with risk of UI progression over 2 years [45]. Although caffeine reduction is part of the interventions recommended as first line treatment of urinary incontinence, based on these results, there is insufficient evidence for discouraging coffee consumption among women with urinary incontinence. At least, these data suggest that consumption of low to moderate doses of caffeine may not have a major impact on the development or worsening of urinary incontinence.

Regarding UI in men, there are data suggesting that caffeine intake is associated with the presence of moderate to severe UI [48]. Thus, the evaluation of caffeine reduction in men with UI is needed.

Several lines of evidence suggest that the chronic consumption of large amounts of cola-based soft drinks may result in severe symptomatic hypokalaemia than clearly predisposes to the development of potentially fatal complications such as cardiac arrhythmias [49,50]. Neurological adverse effects: Seizures occur in either a dose-related or idiosyncratic way in susceptible individuals [51,52]. An excessive intake of diet coke increases the epileptogenic effect of the hiponatremia, and aspartame, a sweetener used in diet coke, is known for its epileptogenic potential. A caffeine intake over 180 mg per day can increase intraocular pressure and produces miosis [4]. Caffeine is a common component of many over the counter headache preparations, and many of us reach for a strong coffee at the onset of "fuzzy headedness" or minor headache. The association between coffee intake and subarachnoid haemorrhage therefore may be one of reverse causality, in which an unidentified nonspecific prodromal symptomatology invokes caffeine intake and therefore the appearance of association with subarachnoid haemorrhage [53]. Psychiatric adverse effects: Symptoms of severe anxiety have been reported with caffeine chronic heavy consumption. There are multiple reports of worsening psychosis related to heavy caffeine intake. Poor sleep in children has been associated with poor school performance, atopy, frequent headaches, and depressive symptoms [12]. In spite of its wide social acceptance, habitual caffeine use typically results in physiologic dependence. Caffeine withdrawal is a well docummented phenomenon, and may be severe enough to cause significant functional impairment [12]. Sleep-disordered-breathing is independently associated with caffeinated soda use in general community [53].

Side Effects in Chronic Exposure [1,4]

There is no wide evidence that moderate consumption of caffeine causes a significant health risk in healthy adults. The effects of chronic high-dose caffeine intake in children and adolescents are unknown [12].

Caffeine intake is not directly related to the risk of hypertension. Despite affects lipid metabolism and endothelial function, there are conflicting published data on the increased risk of coronary heart disease, contributing or in morbidity and mortality.

Caffeine decreases bone density, because it could enhance the action of the glucocorticoid receptor, which is a major risk factor for osteoporosis. Its intake is not demostrated to cause nephropathy. However, is one of the many factors implicated in female urinary incontinence.

There is a clear association of caffeine use with gastric or duodenal ulcers, related with the gastric acid secretion and colonic activity stimulated by caffeine. However, the consumption of coffee exacerbates gastroesophageal reflux, although this effect could be caused by other constituyents of the different coffee caffeine.

Caffeine intake usually causes insomnia; however, in some people, caffeine produces paradoxical sedation, an idiosyncratic phenomenon that has also been described with amphetamine. In contrast, caffeine withdrawal produces hypersomnia.

Caffeine can disturb the functions of cell cycle control and several DNA repair mechanisms, may increase or antagonize exposure and mutagenic potential carcinogens. Although the results are contradictory has suggested a link between coffee consumption and pancreatic cancer. It has been reported that mutation of the K-ras gene, that is a marker for exocrine pancreatic cancer, increases as dose dependently consumption. On the other hand, several studies have linked chronic coffee consumption with reduced risk of colorectal cancer, but no prospective study confirmed this result. Further, the caffeine has suppressive effects on tumor cells in the experimental metastasis [4].

Toxicity

Caffeine overdoses produce multiple symptoms, most of which are commonly associated with a marked increase in adrenergic tone. These can include hypertension, tachycardia, dysrhythmias, and central nervous and skeletal muscle stimulation [12,55].

In people who do not drink coffee, half-life of caffeine is two times greater, which explains the higher incidence of poisoning in this group [4]. Caffeine poisonings also occur in users who increase their dose or habitual heavy users of high doses of caffeine.

When acute caffeine ingestion is suspected, the history should address the following aspects: use of prescription medications or over-the-counter drugs, use of illicit drugs or recent caffeine ingestion or behavior compatible with such ingestión. When ingested in excessive amounts for extended periods, caffeine produces a specific toxidrome (caffeinism), witch combines cardiovascular, neurological and gastrointestinal syntoms [56].

Death is an uncommon result of caffeine poisoning. A separate report published by the FDA's Center for Food Safety and Applied Nutrition and Adverse Event Reporting System cited 16 deaths related to caffeinated energy drinks between 2004 and 2010 were 16 deaths [12,56]. Swedish researchers conducted an extensive analysis defining toxic doses of caffeine. Of 5000 forensic autopsies performed in Sweden each year, 1% had caffeine levels exceeding 10 µg/mL. To place this in perspective, a single cup of standard brewed coffee results in blood caffeine levels of 1 to 2 µg/mL. It is very important to note that alcohol and other medications can prolong the 5-hour half-life of caffeine and contribute to its toxic effects, and that drug interactions may appear. Caffeine and many medications are metabolized via the cytochrome P450 1A2 pathway. Some fatalities might have resulted from heightened and prolonged caffeine levels attributable to multiple drugs being metabolized by the same metabolic pathway. The rate of drug metabolism varies from person to person and depends on body size, age, sex, and genetic factors. Some people may have cardiac or liver diseases that could increase susceptibility to caffeine related adverse effects, making a routinely consumed amount of caffeine more dangerous. Some ingredients in energy drinks may confer toxicity or promote drug interactions [3]. Fatal caffeine overdoses in adults are relatively rare and require the ingestion of a large quantity of the drug, typically in excess of 5 g [1,4,6], that can cause ventricular dysrhythmia. There are reported doses of 5-50 g; recovery after ingestion of 30 g has been reported. Our research group successfully attended two brothers poisoned with 10 g of oral caffein [57]. In general, toxic and fatal reactions have been associated with blood concentrations in excess of 15 and 80 mg/L, respectively. Postmortem redistribution may account for increased caffeine concentrations in heart blood [6].

Children are a special risk of poisoning because the caffeine content of each package with caffeinated energy drink is very high. One study found that an intake of 5 mg/kg body weight leads to elevated blood pressure and lower heart rate, without concomitant changes in energy metabolism in children aged 9-11 years. This amounts to 160 mg caffeine/day in a 10-year-old child weighing 30 kg, which is equivalent to the caffeine content of a single 16-oz Monster or Rockstar energy drink. This is consistent with data from an earlier report by the European Food Safety Authority's (EFSA) Scientific Committee on Food, stating that an intake of 5 mg caffeine/kg body weight is sufficient to increase arousal, irritability, nervousness, and anxiety in children, especially if they do not normally consume caffeine [56]. More research that can guide actions of regulatory agencies is needed to regular caffeinated energy drinks, their supplements and their marketing campaings [12,41].

The Usual Symptoms of Caffeine Intoxication

Symptoms of caffeine intoxication are an exaggeration of their pharmacological effects and include [1,4,56]:

- Central nervous system (CNS) features: Headache, lightheadedness, anxiety, agitation, tremulousness, perioral and extremity tingling, confusion, psychosis, seizures, pupils dilated but reactive to light. In severe patients, coma and death.

- Cardiovascular features: Palpitations or racing heart rate, chest pain, widened pulse pressure, dyrhytmias, hypotension, infarction, heart failure.
- Gastrointestinal features: Nausea and vomiting, abdominal pain, diarrhea, bowel incontinence, anorexia, hyperactive bowel sounds.
- Methabolic features: acidosis, rhabdomyolysis, sweating, hypokalemia,
- Respiratory features: pulmonary edema, tachypnea, hypocapnia.
- Chronic caffeine toxicity may manifest as myopathy, hypokalemia, muscle weakness, nausea, vomiting, diarrhea and weight loss.

Diagnosis

In hemodynamically stable patients with mild symptoms and a clear history of caffeine ingestion, no laboratory studies are indicated. Laboratory studies are indicated in patients with moderate-to-severe symptoms of caffeine toxicity [56]. May be helpful a complete blood analysis and an arterial blood gas analysis; patients with chest pain, palpitations, tachycardia, or an irregular heart rhythm should be evaluated with electrocardiography, and those with fever, chest pain, altered mental status or respiratory complaints, with a chest radiograph.

Serum caffeine concentration determinations do not influence management but could be interesting from a viewpoint of toxicokinetics or ingested dose is unknown.

Management

Prehospital care is primarily supportive, and most cases resolve. Emergency management of more severe cases includes the following: ABCs (*A* irway, *B* reathing, *C* irculation), mangement of hypotension, correction of dysrhythmias, management of seizures (with benzodiazepines or barbiturates), correction of metabolic disturbances (hypokalemia, rhabdomyolysis, hyperglycemia, metabolic acidosis), and treatment of prolonged vomiting [56]. It is also recommended gastric decontamination with actívated charcoal, enhance elimination with sorbitol, hemoperfusion or hemodialysis (if the severity required) [57]. If cardiovascular collapse appears, lidocaine or phenylephrine are indicated to stabilized the patient [55]. In patients with tachyarrhythmia with prolonged Qt interval, amiodarone should be avoided [6].

Table 9. Management of caffeine intoxication

Sing/symptom/goal	Management
Gastric decontamination	Single dose activated charcoal within 1 h of ingestión
Enhance elimination	Hemodialysis (if ventricular dysrrhytmias, severe acidosis, seizures, hypotension, coma, caffeine serum concentration > 90µg/ml)
Nausea, vomiting	Ondasetron
Hypokalemia	Correction typically no necessary unless dysrrhythmia present
Central nervous system excitation	Benzodiazepines
Seizures	Benzodiazepines. If refractory considerer: barbiturates, propofol.
Tachycardia	Intravenous fluids, benzodiazepines. Considerer beta adrenergic antagonists in ventricular dysrhythmias or calcium cannel antagonists
Hypotension	Intravenous fluids. If no response: phenylephrine or lidocaine.

Coffee Consumption and Mortality

Coffee consumption has been linked to various beneficial and detrimental health effects, but data on its relation with mortality are sparse [56]. In a recent retrospective study of 43.727 subjects who were followed for a median of 17 years, heavy coffee consumption, defined as more than 28 cups (8 oz.) per week, was associated with an increased risk of all-cause mortality among men. For men and women 55 years of age and younger, the association between heavy coffee consumption and all-cause mortality was more pronounced [56]. In a multivariate analysis, men who drank more than 28 cups of coffee had a significant 21% increased risk of all-cause mortality. In women, there was no statistically significant difference in the risk of all-cause mortality. In men younger than 55 years, drinking more than 28 cups per week was associated with a 56% increased risk of death in comparison with nondrinkers. In women younger than 55 years, such heavy consumption increased the risk of death by

113% in comparison with those who did not drink coffee. Overall, there was no association between coffee consumption and cardiovascular mortality.

Despite these results, in another study including two large cohorts (41.736 men and 86.214 women), reserchers did not found a detrimental effect of coffee consumption on mortality [57] in either cohort. In addition, regular coffee consumption was associated with lower risk of death, mainly in women. Those findings are consistent with the possible beneficial effects of coffee on inflammation, endothelial function, and risk for type 2 diabetes, with a moderately reduction of cardiovascular disease mortality risk. By contrast, coffee consumption was not statistically significantly associated with risk for cancer death after adjustment for potential confounders. Decaffeinated coffee consumption was also associated with a small reduction in all-cause and cardiovascular disease mortality. The main limitation in this study was than coffee consumption was estimated from selfreport.

The conclusion we can draw, in view of what has been said, is that caffeine consumption should be in moderation.

5. IMPACT ON PERFORMANCE, MOOD AND SPORTS

Dr. S. Castaño, RN. N. Ruiz and Dr. E. Corral

Many researchers think that people who don't use caffeine regularly and who haven't developed a dependence on it, usually become significantly more alert and better able to perform cognitive and motor tasks if they're given the right dose of caffeine they use caffeine regularly. However its benefits on performance are unclear. For example, in 2005, researchers gave 96 regular caffeine users a battery of tests after two weeks on and two weeks off caffeine. The participants did no better when they were consuming caffeine than when they weren't.

Habitual caffeine users feel good about caffeine due to the alleviation of withdrawal symptoms. If they have a cup of coffee or a caffeinated energy drink, the symptoms disappear and they feel much better again.

Impact on Performance

Coffee and beverages containing coffee consumption is linked to the stimulant properties of caffeine. Caffeine increases feelings of alertness, fights fatigue and generally provides a sense of wellbeing [4,59]; Caffeine consumption leads to increased ability to concentrate, particularly when subjects are fatigued or working at night [60], like emergency medicine residents, whose high prevalence of caffeine use may explain the low prevalence of prescription psychostimulants [61]. Caffeine is inexpensive, familiar, and effective at increasing alertness and is easily available without prescription.

Caffeine is used to mitigate the fatigue experienced during the circadian adaptation associated with the normal circadian nadir that corresponds to times of wakefulness and performance at the destination. The strategic use of caffeine [eg, 50-mg to 200-mg pill or beverage] in combination with a 15-minute to 30-minute nap has been shown to be effective in improving cognitive function in sleep-deprived states and at the circadian nadir [62]. A systematic review of 13 randomized trials of persons with jet lag or shift work disorder found that caffeine significantly improved concept formation, reasoning, memory, orientation, attention, and perception when compared to placebo [60]. In high doses and in certain individuals, may occur not very nice effects, such as anxiety.

A double-blind, placebo-controlled study [59] with individuals having several regimes caffeine, showed it led to to increased alertness and anxiety and improved performance on simple and choice reactive tasks, a cognitive vigilance task, a task requiring sustained response and a dual task involving tracking and target detection.

Mechanism

The molecular targets responsible for the behavioral effects of caffeine and have been extensively investigated in rodents. It is mainly due to blockade of adenosine receptors, but the relative role of each subtype is still being investigated. The dopaminergic system seems to be involved. Most of the central effects of caffeine on concentrations found in beverages is due to the blockade of adenosine receptors. The anxiolytic effects of a xanthine with extended ring and containing an arylpiperazine component seems to be due to the agonistic activity on serotonin receptors [4].

Caffeine Consumption in Sports

The ergogenic effects of caffeine on athletic performance have been shown in many studies. It is well established than lower doses can be as effective as higher doses during exercise performance without any negative coincidence; after a period of cessation, restarting caffeine intake at a low amount before performance can provide the same ergogenic effects as acute intake; caffeine can be taken gradually at low doses to avoid tolerance during the course of 3 or 4 days, just before intense training to sustain exercise intensity; and caffeine can improve cognitive aspects of performance, such as concentration, when an athlete has not slept well [63]. Caffeine also reduces the perception of muscle pain [50] and the perception of how hard we are working, which makes us feel better when exercising and may help us exercise longer.

Caffeine can improve physical performance in endurance exercise like running, but the effect is less for short bursts of movement such as lifting weights or sprinting [63]. In sprint and power events that rely mainly on the phosphogen system (<10 seconds), caffeine improved peak power output, speed, and isokinetic strength; however, in events that heavily rely on the glycolytic system (15 seconds to 3 minutes), no improvements were found with caffeine use, and in fact, it may have been detrimental to performance during repeated bouts of exercise [63].

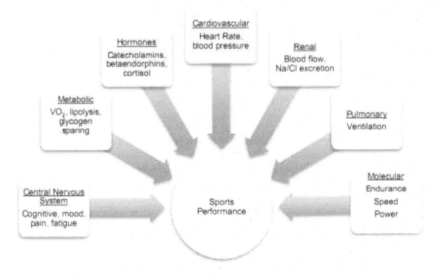

Figure 2. Effects of caffeine on body systems and sports performance [63, modiffied].

Ingestion of a caffeinated sports drink increases urine production, and this diuretic effect is also observed when a caffeinated beverage is used after exercise. However, during submaximal prolonged exercise, several studies coincide on that the addition of caffeine to a sports drink does not significantly increase urine production.

Mechanism

The stimulation of the sympathetic nervous system by caffeine acts on multiple metabolic pathways to improve endurance performance; until recent years the suspicion was than it helps the body to burn more of its ample stores of fat instead of the limited stores of carbohydrate that are in our muscles. Recently Davis et al. proposed a mechanism by which caffeine delays fatigue through its effects on the central nervous system, where it stimulant through its action as an adenosin receptor antagonist, and its alangesic effects on central nervous system[63]. It leads to a release of Ca^{++} from skeletal muscle sarcoplasmic reticulum, an increase of lipolysis by a modest raise of muscle glycogen, and by the indirect increase in catecholamine release [50,63], witch causes transient elevation in blood pressure [40].

However, in repeated bouts of maximal exercise that last 15 seconds to 3 minutes and thus rely heavily on anaerobic glycolysis, caffeine has been clearly shown to have no effect or to be a negative factor in power and sprint performance, possibly because of an increase in plasma ammonia levels and a decrease in intracellular pH [63].

Practical Applications of Caffeine for Athletes [63]

Nonusing athletes who are considering caffeine as an ergogenic aid will be unaccustomed to its cognitive and physiologic effects, and they should test its effects before implementing a caffeine strategy for training or competition. If an athlete decides to stop consuming caffeine before competition to increase its ergogenic effects during competition, he or she should reduce gradually caffeine consumption at least 1 week before competition to be completely free from withdrawal effects.

Caffeine ingestión (i.e. 4.5 mg/kg) can benefit high-volume or intense endurance training. Caffeine should be ingested, at the latest, 3 hours before power, sprint, and short endurance events or 1 hour before prolonged endurance events. Acute redosing with caffeine does not necessarily improve performance; however, if the events are more than 6 hours apart, it may be beneficial.

Because caffeine increases plasma lactate levels and decreases intracellular pH, it may be contraindicated for athletes in sprint events that last 30 seconds to 3 minutes.

In chronic consumers (3 and 6 mg/kg/d), acute caffeine ingestion did not alter fluid–electrolyte and physiologic responses during exercise in heat (37.7° C), when compared to a placebo. The effects of ingesting caffeine with a carbohydrate solution, with an amino acid solution, and during creatine loading require further study.

6. PSYCHIATRIC DISORDERS RELATED TO CAFFEINE CONSUMPTION

Dr. M. Prieto, Dr. B. Fernández-Miret and Dr. G. Balziskueta

Introduction

Caffeine is a xanthine with antagonistic effect on the adenosine receptor that works as a CNS stimulant. It is found naturally in more than 60 plants (coffee, tea, cocoa...). It can be consumed from different sources and consumer products. Coffee, tea, chocolate and cola soft drinks are the main sources of caffeine, which is consumed at almost all ages and socioeconomic strata. Coffee is the main contributor of caffeine in adult diet. Today about 80-90% of the Western population ingests caffeine daily. It is the most widely used psychostimulant in the world with an average intake per person of 200 mg/day (2-3 cups of coffee) approximately. In addition, it has been described that 20 to 30% of Americans consume more than 500 mg/day of caffeine [64]. Among patients with mental disorders, this percentage is much higher [65].

Caffeine has a competitive antagonist effect on adenosine A1 and A2A receptors [66]. It works as a CNS stimulant in a way that in low-moderate consumption of caffeine (<400 mg/day) produces a dose-dependent activation of widespread CNS. This increases alertness, reduces tiredness and fatigue, produces a slight feeling of well-being, increases the ability to maintain an intellectual effort and maintains wakefulness despite sleep deprivation. The possible adverse effects of caffeine in moderate doses are few and without potential danger. Among the most common are anxiety, irritability, insomnia and gastrointestinal irritation. But it can also cause palpitations, tachycardia, tremor and nervousness. High doses can provoke intense anxiety, fear and panic attacks.

Neurobiological Basis

The adenosinic antagonism of caffeine is the fundamental mechanism by which exerts its stimulant effects[67]. Adenosine is a inhibitory neurotransmitter in the CNS. Adenosine receptors are widely distributed throughout the CNS and present in critical structures for the implementation of cognitive abilities such as the hippocampus, the cerebral cortex, the cerebellum and the thalamus. The blockade of adenosine receptors prevents the union of the adenosine and its inhibitory action. This results in moderate increases in the activity of neurotransmitter systems that have adenosine receptors such as the noradrenergic, cholinergic, dopaminergic and serotoninergic [66,68]. Stimulation of noradrenergic and cholinergic systems has been linked to increases in alertness, attention and ability to process new information, being this particularly evident in deficit situations and states of sleep deprivation [69]. The noradrenergic system also would be related to some symptoms of caffeine withdrawal. The action on the dopaminergic activity would be the mechanism associated with the caffeine implication on the brain reward systems responsible for reinforcement and addiction. This mechanism could facilitate patterns of abuse and dependence of caffeine. Nevertheless the changes produced in dopaminergic activity should be much higher than the one who produces caffeine, even at high doses administered. This hypothesis of dopaminergic hyperactivity supports the clinical findings that associate caffeine intake with an exacerbation of psychotic symptoms in subjects with schizophrenia [20]. Finally, activation of the serotonergic system is related to the potential benefits of caffeine on mood. Caffeine can induce positive mood effects but these effects are modest. The administration of caffeine in more severe clinical circumstances, such as major depression, is an insufficient therapeutic strategy to reverse the symptoms of the patients.

Caffeine-Related Psychiatric Disorders

Caffeine-related psychiatric disorders have not been included in international diagnostic classifications for mental disorders until recently. It is in the DSM-III (1980) where caffeine intoxication is incorporated for the first time as a diagnostic cathegory. In the DSM-IV (1994) and current DSM-IV-TR (2000) has been remained caffeine intoxication and has been included caffeine withdrawal as a disorder, classified in the Appendix B "Criteria Sets and Axes Provided for Further Study". In international diagnostic classifications for mental disorders is not yet accepted the caffeine dependence disorder. According to the DSM-IV-TR Diagnostic Manual for mental disorders, currently, data are insufficient to determine if the described symptoms of abuse or dependence on caffeine are associated with a "clinically significant impairment" that met the diagnostic criteria for substance dependence. In this manual, the caffeine-induced disorders include caffeine-induced anxiety disorder, caffeine-induced sleep disorder and unspecified caffeine-induced disorder. According to the DSM-IV-TR is unknown the real prevalence of caffeine-related disorders.

There is no evidence that chronic exposure to typical daily dose of caffeine in healthy adults may entail a significant risk for the health. However, different symptoms and psychiatric disorders have been associated with caffeine consumption: it can induce or exacerbate anxiety and panic attacks, influence in mood, precipitate psychotic symptoms, cause sleep disorders and behave as a substance of abuse, with specific diagnostic criteria for intoxication, positive reinforcing properties possibility, risk of development of tolerance phenomena and, in case of a sudden interruption, has been described the presence of a specific withdrawal syndrome.

a) Anxiety and Anxiety Disorders

Caffeine can cause anxiety symptoms in normal individuals and in those with pre-existing anxiety disorders [70]. Patients with panic disorder and performance social anxiety disorder seem to be particulary sensitive to anxiogenic effects of caffeine [69]. In the DSM-IV-TR anxiety disorder induced by caffeine is included as a diagnostic category with specific diagnostic criteria. The essential feature of the disorder is the presence of prominent anxiety symptoms that are considered secondary to the direct physiological effects of the substance.

b) Mood and Mood Disorders

Caffeine has been shown both, to induce mood changes, particularly at higher doses, and to protect from mood symptoms at moderate doses. Moderate caffeine intake can induce positive mood effects [69]. Caffeine cessation over a couple of days may increase anxiety and depression scores

[71]. However its putative therapeutic effects on depression have been insufficiently studied.

A few case reports have also suggested that caffeine can induce mania [72] and that excessive caffeine intake may hamper the recovery of patients with bipolar disorder or manic-type mood episodes [73]. Expert opinion and guidelines for the treatment of bipolar disorder recommend discontinuation of caffeine intake as one of the first steps in the treatment of mania.

c) Sleep Disorders Induced by Caffeine

It is a diagnosis included in the DSM-IV-TR. The essential feature of this disorder is the presence of sleep disturbances as a result of consumption or cessation of the substance. Caffeine related sleep disorder typically involves insomnia although some individuals coinciding with the period of abstinence may refer hypersomnia and daytime sleepiness. Caffeine exerts a dose-dependent effect, as consumption increases wakefulness is increased and sleep continuity is decreased. Polysomnographic records show a greater sleep latency and increased wakefulness.

d) Pyschosis and Psychotic Symptoms

As a competitive adenosine antagonist caffeine affects dopaminergic transmission and has been reported that caffeine can induce psychosis in healthy subjects ingesting caffeine at high doses [74] and worsen psychotic symptoms in individuals with psychotic disorders [75].

Caffeine intake may be higher in patients with schizophrenia or at least in a subgroup of them [65].

Caffeine as a Substance of Abuse

Caffeine Intoxication

Acute or chronic over-consumption of caffeine can produce a caffeine-poisoning syndrome. The symptoms are an exaggeration of its pharmacological effects [76]. The most common clinical symptoms are alterations at the CNS as nervousness, restlessness, anxiety, excitement, racing thoughts, sleep disturbances, increased motor activity, irritability and mood changes. Simultaneously, tend to produce other somatic manifestations such as palpitations, tachycardia, facial flushing, diaphoresis, tremor, diuresis, gastrointestinal disturbance, muscle twitching and cardiac arrhythmias. The consumption of more than 1 gram of caffeine can produce verbiage, confused thinking, arrhythmias, severe agitation, tinnitus and mild visual hallucinations (light flashes). Acute doses above 10 grams of caffeine can cause generalized tonic clonic seizures, respiratory failure and death [75]. There is no a well-defined dose of caffeine from which may develop poisoning symptoms in general population. Although, according to available data, it can be expected that the risk of developing clinical manifestations is high when the daily caffeine intake exceeds 500-600 mg. Nevertheless caffeine intoxication may not appear despite the consumption of large amounts of caffeine due to the development of tolerance [77].

The DSM-IV^{TM} specifies the criteria for the diagnosis of caffeine intoxication (Table 10).

Table 10. Caffeine Intoxication diagnostic criteria. From: Caffeine-related disorders. In: American Psychiatric Association: *Diagnostic and Statistical Manual of Mental Disorders*, Fourth Edition. Washington, DC, American Psychiatric Association, 1994. p. 213

Diagnostic criteria for 305.90 Caffeine Intoxication
A. Recent consumption of caffeine, usually in excess of 250 mg (e.g., more than 2-3 cups of brewed coffee).   B. Five (or more) of the following signs, developing during, or shortly after, caffeine use: (1) restlessness   (2) nervousness   (3) excitement   (4) insomnia   (5) flushed face   (6) diuresis   (7) gastrointestinal disturbance   (8) muscle twitching   (9) rambling flow of thought and speech   (10) tachycardia or cardiac arrhythmia   (11) periods of inexhaustibility   (12) psychomotor agitation   C. The symptoms in Criterion B cause clinically significant distress or impairment in social, occupational, or other important areas of functioning.   D. The symptoms are not due to a general medical condition and are not better accounted for by another mental disorder (e.g., an Anxiety Disorder)

Caffeine Dependence

The essential feature of substance dependence consists on a cluster of cognoscitive, behavioural and physiological symptoms indicating that the individual continues consuming the substance despite the emergence of significant problems related to it.

Current classification systems for mental disorders do not recognize the existence of the disorder by caffeine dependence. However clinical evidence supports this diagnosis in some individuals with problematic use of caffeine. In a study Strain et al. provide evidence of the possible existence of a syndrome of caffeine dependence [78]. They show as up to 59% of adults in the study met a sufficient number of diagnostic criteria for dependence of the DSM-IV-TR: development of tolerance after continued use, specific withdrawal symptoms following cessation of consumption, persistent efforts to reduce or stop consumption and continued use despite knowledge of the harmful effects of the substance.

In addition, caffeine has a positive enhancer effect since regular use at low-moderate doses produced subjective effects that are generally classified as pleasant or enjoyable, leading to the maintenance of consumption. Nevertheless it has been suggested that this mechanism of self-administration may be more as a result of the search for relief from the withdrawal symptoms (after the night without consumption) than the positive reinforcing effects of caffeine itself. Anyway, the reinforcement mechanism of caffeine is different and underpowered compared to other psychostimulants such as cocaine or amphetamine [79].

Tolerance

It is defined as the need for increased amounts of the substance to achieve the desired effect or as the effect of the same amount of substance clearly decreases with continued use.

There are few studies on caffeine tolerance. It is generally accepted that caffeine tolerance at the level of the CNS is less when compared with other effects such as diuresis. It is difficult to assess whether the lack of effects on consumers of average doses of coffee is the development of tolerance or due to interindividual differences in susceptibility to xanthines. Several studies have shown that regular consumption of high doses of coffee produces effects that are not completely suppressed by the development of tolerance since the accumulation of caffeine in the body follows a non-linear model [80].

Caffeine Withdrawal Syndrome

Characteristic withdrawal syndrome appears secondary to abrupt cessation or reduction in consumption of caffeine-containing products in individuals who previously took it regularly. In several controlled studies is described as a real phenomenon and the DSM-IV-TR facilitates research criteria for caffeine withdrawal (Table 11).

Table 11. Research criteria for caffeine withdrawal. From: Criteria Sets and Axes Provided for Furder Study: Caffeine Whithdrawal. In: American Psychiatric Association: *Diagnostic and Statistical Manual of Mental Disorders*, Fourth Edition. Washington, DC, American Psychiatric Association, 1994. p. 709

Research criteria for caffeine withdrawal

A. Prolonged daily use of caffeine.
B. Abrupt cessation of caffeine use, or reduction in the amount of caffeine used, closely followed by headache and one (or more) of the following symptoms:

(1) marked fatigue or drowsiness
(2) marked anxiety or depression
(3) nausea or vomiting

C. The symptoms in Criterion B cause clinically significant distress or impairment in social, occupational, or other important areas of functioning.
D. The symptoms are not due to the direct physiological effects of a general medical condition (e.g., migraine, viral illness) and are not better accounted for by another mental disorder.

Caffeine withdrawal syndrome is mainly characterized by headache, dizziness, mild hypothymia, irritability, anxiety, tiredness and fatigue. Other symptoms that may occur are difficulty of concentration, decreased alertness, decreased performance, lower sociability, nausea, craving, yawning, irritability, muscle tension and motor slowness. According to a comprehensive review [81], the most common symptoms of caffeine withdrawal are headache and fatigue.

Several epidemiological studies have described caffeine withdrawal symptoms by 50 % to 70 % of studied caffeine consumers [82]. In a controlled double-blind study versus placebo symptoms of abrupt withdrawal of caffeine were studied and it was found that 52% have moderate or severe degree of headache and up to 11% have depressive and anxiety symptoms [83]. In another retrospective population-based study 27% of the daily caffeine users reported headache, fatigue and dizziness if abstinent over than 24 hours [84].

While it is estimated that the dose of regular consumption necessary to allow a withdrawal syndrome to caffeine is around 500 - 600 mg/day, controlled studies have shown that people with lower consumption may have withdrawal symptoms too [83]. Therefore, although this syndrome has a higher prevalence among individuals with high consumption, it may occur also in individuals with much lower consumption. The number and severity of withdrawal symptoms correlate with the amount of caffeine and the abruptness of withdrawal. In general, the symptoms are more severe as the daily dose that stops consuming is greater.

Withdrawal symptoms tend to start 12-24 hours after the last consumption, with a peak at 24-48 hours and lasting up to one week. These symptoms are time-limited and reversible after restarting caffeine intake[85]. In different experimental studies it has been demonstrated the emergence of withdrawal symptoms with the cessation of caffeine, that disappear or are alleviated by consuming it again.

Comorbidity

Individuals with caffeine-related disorders are most likely to present additional disorders related to substance use than subjects without this diagnosis. In addition, about 2/3 of large daily amounts of caffeine consumers also consume sedatives and hypnotics [82]. A high proportion of consumers of high doses of caffeine also take benzodiazepines.

The multivariate structural equation models of caffeine, tobacco and alcohol consumption indicate that a common genetic factor underlies the use of the three substances [82]. Smokers consume more caffeine than non-smokers (either by a common genetic vulnerability or by associated with increased elimination of caffeine in smokers). The intense consumption and alcohol dependence is thus associated itself to intense consumption and a pattern of caffeine dependence.

Several studies have shown the daily intake of high doses of caffeine in psychiatric patients (up to an average of 5 or more cups of coffee a day).

7. CAFFEINE IN MEDICINE. DRUG INTERACTIONS

Dr. H. Barrasa, Dr. S. Cabañes and Dr. F. Fonseca

INTRODUCTION

Caffeine acts as a non-selective adenosine receptor antagonist in the central nervous system. Its main effects are as psychostimulant, analgesic, acting in addition on the respiratory, muscular and cardiovascular systems [1]. According to its multiple effects in the human organism, caffeine has been used in the treatment of different conditions and it has been associated with multiple beneficial and deleterious effects, as well.

Caffeine as Treatment

Psychostimulant

Caffeine produced a dose dependent widespread activation of CNS, possibly by increasing the release of norepinephrine. Increases alertness, reduces tiredness and fatigue, increases the ability to maintain an intellectual effort and maintains wakefulness despite sleep deprivation.

Apnea of Prematurity

Caffeine is the respiratory stimulant of choice for the treatment of apnea [86]. It increases the sensitivity of bulbar respiratory center to carbon dioxide, stimulates respiratory central drive and increases the contraction of skeletal muscles, improving diaphragmatic contractility. The prevention of apnea may occur through competitive inhibition of adenosine.

The international, randomized, placebo- controlled Caffeine for Apnea of Prematurity trial has shown that caffeine therapy reduces the duration of exposure to positive airway pressure and supplemental oxygen and the rates of neonatal morbidities, including bronchopulmonary dysplasia and severe retinopathy of prematurity; improves the rate of survival without neurodevelopmental impairment at 18 to 21 months of age; and is cost-effective [26,87].

Dosage: the starting dose of caffeine citrate 20mg/kg is followed by a maintenance dose of 5mg/kg, beginning 24 hours after the loading dose. These doses may be administered orally or by infusion for 30min IV (loading dose) and 10min (maintenance dose).

Sleep Deprivation and Fatigue

For sleepiness and fatigue, caffeine has been the most widely used CNS stimulant. Although we know its chemistry and part of the mechanism of action (a nonselective adenosine receptor antagonist) it is still not generally recommended because its short half life, tolerance development, and it still only targets symptoms, not the underlying etiology [88].

Despite its limitations, it is useful in some situations. Caffeine has been evaluated in simulated shift-work conditions. Caffeine (300 mg) increased performance and alertness in a simulated night-shift setting and in shift workers on the night shift. Caffeine administration is thought to diminish the influence of homeostatic sleep drive and thus improve physiologic alertness and some cognitive-performance measures during extended wakefulness and circadian misalignment [89-91].

Jet Lag and Travel Fatigue

Caffeine is used to mitigate the fatigue experienced during the circadian adaptation associated with the normal circadian nadir that corresponds to times of wakefulness and performance at the destination. The strategic use of caffeine (50-mg to 200-mg pill or beverage) in combination with a 15-minute to 30-minute nap has been shown to be effective in improving cognitive function in sleep-deprived states and at the circadian nadir [92].

Use in Sports

There have been numerous positive reports of the improvements of caffeine on mood, mental alertness, decreased tiredness, and energetic arousal [93,94]. The ergogenic effectiveness and cognitive symptoms of caffeine are represented by an inverted dose– response curve and a varying time course depending on age, gender, and body size.

Caffeine is widely used among athletes. There are some recommendations to consider the global effects of caffeine on the body: Lower doses can be as effective as higher doses during exercise performance without any negative coincidence; after a period of cessation, restarting caffeine intake at a low amount before performance can provide the same ergogenic effects as acute intake; caffeine can be taken gradually at low doses to avoid tolerance during the course of 3 or 4 days, just before intense training to sustain exercise intensity; and caffeine can improve cognitive aspects of performance, such as concentration, when an athlete has not slept well. Athletes and coaches also must consider how a person's body size, age, gender, previous use, level of tolerance, and the dose itself all influence the ergogenic effects of caffeine on sports performance [63].

Parkinson´s Disease (PD)

Lifelong caffeine use has been consistently associated with lower risk of PD in prospective studies (compared with non–coffee drinkers, relative risk of Parkinson's disease was 0.69 (95% CI, 0.59–0.80) for coffee drinkers [95]). Moreover, a recent clinical trial showed that caffeine provided only equivocal borderline improvement in excessive somnolence in PD, but improved objective motor measures. However, these findings must be confirmed in separate longer-term trials explicitly designed to assess these effects [96].

Effect on Alzheimer's disease: There are few studies examining the relationship between coffee and Alzheimer disease. In a pooled analysis of two cohort and two case control studies on coffee and Alzheimer disease, coffee consumption was associated with a small protective effect against this disease (relative risk [RR] 0.70, 95% CI 0.55-0.90) [2,97].

Analgesic

Caffeine possesses some analgesic effects. These are due partly to its adjuvant potency to potentiate the analgesic properties of other medications. Numerous widely consumed combination medications marketed for the reliefing of headache symptoms include caffeine as an essential component. Caffeine can increase the plasma area under the curve (AUC) and Cmax of acetaminophen or aspirin, as well as decrease the plasma clearance of acetaminophen [98,99].

Caffeine also has intrinsic acute analgesic properties. With respect to headache, these analgesic effects are of modest magnitude and can be generalized to several different headache disorders. There are few controlled prospective randomized studies, but there seem to indicate an analgesic efficacy in the treatment of tension headache and migraine without aura, as well as increase and prolong the analgesic effect of paracetamol by the pharmacodynamic interaction. For the relief of tension-type or migraine headache, randomized trials indicate that oral caffeine dosages of 200 mg or more are required [100]. In a controlled trial [101], 300 mg of oral caffeine produced statistically significant headache relief within 4 hours of postdural puncture headache (PDPH) onset. However, a recent Cochrane Review concluded that although intravenous caffeine has demonstrated efficacy for

PDPH in patients who have received spinal anesthesia, its efficacy and safety remain uncertain in patients presenting to the emergency department after a typical diagnostic lumbar puncture [4,102].

Moreover, caffeine has potential advantages in patients on chronic morphine therapy limited by the incidence of side effects, the risk of dependence and withdrawal, although it may be useful to improve cognitive performance in cancer patients treated with morphine. It may potentially be useful for its effects on gastrointestinal activity and there is evidence that it increases the analgesic effect of nonopioids. Further studies are necessary to evaluate whether higher doses of caffeine may be more effective and to establish the role of tolerance to caffeine in this group of patients [103].

On the other hand, it is important to underline that although infrequent intake of caffeine may act as an analgesic for headache or an adjuvant for the actions of other analgesics, with chronic repetitive intake, caffeine is associated with an increased risk of development of analgesic-overuse headache, chronic daily headache and physical dependency. Cessation of caffeine use following chronic exposures leads to a withdrawal syndrome, with headache as a dominant symptom [104].

Determination of Liver Function

Caffeine has been proposed as an ideal test substance for assessing hepatic function, as it is rapidly and completely absorbed after oral intake and it is metabolized primarily by the hepatic cytochrome P-450 dependent mixed function oxidase system. It has been suggested that caffeine concentrations in the plasma after an overnight fast [105] or else plasma concentrations determined 12 h after an oral caffeine load [106] might serve as a simple guide to the severity of hepatic dysfunction.

Moreover, it has been shown that plasma caffeine clearance is significantly reduced in patients with cirrhosis and its elimination half-life is significantly prolonged [107]. In patients with liver cirrhosis, Perlik et al. [108] found significantly lower paraxanthine/caffeine ratio that correlates with lowered elimination of caffeine. Its evaluation enables non-invasive assessment of liver metabolic function from a single sample of saliva.

On the other hand, something to consider is that Cheng et al. [109] in their study showed that cafeine exhibits dose-dependent pharmacokinetics, particularly in subjects with caffeine clearance greater than 1ml/min/kg after a low dose (70mg) of cafeine. These findings imply that if caffeine is to be used as a guide to deteriorating liver function, serial caffeine clearance estimations should be performed in each individual subject, with use of the same dose of caffeine each time.

In any case, although caffeine loading tests are inexpensive, simple to perform and safe, this procedure has not yet been standardized and more comprehensive studies are needed to determine their role in the study of liver function.

Possible Beneficial Effects

Cardiovascular

Coronary Artery Disease

Habitual coffee consumption could potentially reduce the risk of stroke by increasing insulin sensitivity and reducing inflammation. Furthermore, the phenolic compounds of coffee have antioxidant properties and may improve endothelial function. However, whether coffee consumption affects the risk of stroke is unclear. Epidemiological studies of coffee consumption in relation to stroke incidence or mortality have yielded inconsistent results.

There have been developed numerous studies in order to examine the association between coffee consumption and incidence of stroke. Recently, Motofsky et al. conducted a systematic review and a dose-response meta-analysis of prospective studies that assessed the relationship between habitual coffee consumption and the risk of heart failure [110]. They concluded that moderate coffee consumption is inversely associated with risk of heart failure, with the largest inverse association observed for consumption of 4 servings per day.

In addition to the caffeine´s diuretic effect, its natriuretic effect could be used to treat edema associated with congestive heart failure.

Metabolic

Diabetes Mellitus

Coffee intake may improve glucose tolerance via activation of energy metabolism and enhancement of insulin sensitivity and β-cell function, although much of the molecular mechanism remains unknown. Prospective studies have documented an inverse association between coffee consumption and type 2 diabetes risk, especially in women [111,112].

Gastrointestinal

Gallstone Disease

Metabolic studies have shown that coffee affects several hepatobiliary processes that are involved in cholesterol lithogenesis. It has been described a possible protective effect of caffeine intake on the development of gallstones. Women in the Nurses' Health Study who drank two to three cups of regular coffee a day were about 20 percent less likely to be diagnosed with gallstones over a 20-year period than women who drank no regular coffee [113]. Men in the Health Professionals Follow-Up Study who drank two to three cups of regular coffee a day were 40 percent less likely to be diagnosed with gallstones [114].

In both studies, decaf drinkers had no lower risk. However, this protective effect has not been confirmed in subsequent studies [115], so more studies are needed to confirm this association.

Drug Interactions [116]

The polycyclic aromatic hydrocarbon-inducible cytochrome P450 (CYP) 1A2 participates in the metabolism of caffeine as well as of a number of clinically important drugs.

The concentration of caffeine may decrease if its metabolism is induced. Among the inducers are cigars, charred meat, some vegetables, low body mass index, male and habitual coffee consumption itself, as the use of rifampicin, benzodiazepines, carbamazepine, phenobarbital, and omeprazole. The cigar induces the metabolism of caffeine and thus decreasing plasma concentrations. Smokers who consume coffee and stop smoking, may have symptoms of caffeine intoxication, because it doubles its concentration in the absence of smoking.

The concentrations of caffeine may increase with inhibition of its metabolism. This occurs in late pregnancy, in female patients with liver disease and obesity, intake of certain foods and alcohol, and the use of certain medications such as antifungal (fluconazole, ketoconazole), antiarrhythmic drugs (diltiazem, verapamil), antidepressants (paroxetine, fluoxetine, fluvoxamine), antipsychotics (clozapine, olanzapine), methylxanthines (theophylline), oral contraceptives, cimetidine, quinolones and allopurinol.

Some drugs cause an increase in the effect and toxicity of caffeine. They are: quinolones (especially ciprofloxacin and ofloxacin) and CYP1A2 inhibitors such as ketoconazole and fluvoxamine.

Caffeine may reduce sedative and anxiolytic effects of benzodiazepines and barbiturates. Increases the absorption and bioavailability of paracetamol, acetylsalicylic acid and ergotamine. Decreases theophylline clearance and competitively inhibits the metabolism of clozapine, may increase plasma concentrations and the probability of the emergence of adverse effects.

Caffeine produces an additive analgesic effect when administered simultaneously, especially with NSAIDs. In combination with paroxetine may cause serotonin syndrome. Furthermore, caffeine powers stimulants effects of nicotine and may also increases teratogenic effects of alcohol, nicotine and vasoconstrictors.

Low doses of caffeine appear to inhibit, in some experimental models, the antinociceptive effect of various agents such as amitriptyline, venlafaxine, carbamazepine and paracetamol. That seems to be related to the blockade of adenosine receptors A1 type, having an antinociceptive effect. This effect seems to be also important in acupuncture analgesia related and TENS, and theoretically could be inhibited by caffeine.

ABOUT THE AUTHORS

Dr. Sergio Castaño Ávila, Senior house officer, Intensive Care Medicine Department. Álava University Hospital. Registered Nurse. Certificate of Proficiency in Academic Research in Surgery, Medical University of the Basque Country. Assistant profesor in School of Nursing University of Vitoria. Associate professor "Hospital Virtual Miguel Gutierrez", Medical University of the Basque Country.
Email: sergio.castanoavila@osakidetza.net
Dr. Alejandro Martín López, Senior house officer, Intensive Care Medicine Department. Álava University Hospital. Certificate of Proficiency in Academic Research in Surgery, Medical University of the Basque Country. Associate professor "Hospital Virtual Miguel Gutierrez", Medical University of the Basque Country.
RN. Elena Montial Fenández. Graduate in Nursing. Emergencies, Álava University Hospital.
Dr. Miguel Iturbe Rementería, Senior house officer, Intensive Care Medicine Department, Álava University Hospital. Degree in nutrition and dietetics.

Associate professor "Hospital Virtual Miguel Gutierrez", Medical University of the Basque Country.

Dr. Amaia Quintano Rodero. Senior house officer, Intensive Care Medicine Department, Álava University Hospital.

Dr. Borja Fernández Miret Senior house officer, Intensive Care Medicine Department, Álava University Hospital. Certificate of Proficiency in Academic Research in Surgery, Medical University of the Cantabria. Associate professor "Hospital Virtual Miguel Gutierrez", Medical University of the Basque Country.

Dr. Maider Prieto Etxebeste. Senior house officer, Mental Health Center, Barakaldo. Certificate of Proficiency in Academic Research in Neurosciences, Medical University of the Basque Country. Forensic Psychiatric Specialist, UNED.

Dr. Helena Barrasa González, Senior house officer, Intensive Care Medicine Department, Álava University Hospital. Master´s degree in pharmacology. Development, assessment and rational use of medicines. University of Basque Country, Spain.

RN. Estibaliz Jiménez Gutiérrez. Graduate in Nursing, Midwive specialist. Álava University Hospital.

Dr Francisco Javier Maynar Moliner. Clinical Chief. Intensive Care Medicine Department, Álava University Hospital. Associate professor "Hospital Virtual Miguel Gutiérrez", Medical University of the Basque Country.

RN. Nagore Ruiz Cañas. Graduate in Nursing. Nursing Oncology Specialist. Sports Medical Services, Vitoria.

Dr. E. Corral Lozano. Senior house officer, Intensive Care Medicine Department, Álava University Hospital. Associate professor "Hospital Virtual Miguel Gutierrez", Medical University of the Basque Country.

Dr. Goiatz Balziskueta Flórez. Senior house officer, Intensive Care Medicine Department, Álava University Hospital. Associate professor "Hospital Virtual Miguel Gutierrez", Medical University of the Basque Country.

Dr. Sara Cabañes Daro-Francés. Senior house officer, Intensive Care Medicine Department, Álava University Hospital. Associate professor "Hospital Virtual Miguel Gutierrez", Medical University of the Basque Country.

Dr. Fernando Fonseca San Miguel. Head of Intensive Care Medicine Department. Álava University Hospital. Associate professor "Hospital Virtual Miguel Gutiérrez", Medical University of the Basque Country.

REFERENCES

[1] Pardo *Lozano* R, Alvarez García Y, Barral Tafalla D, Farré Albaladejo M. *Cafeína : un nutriente, un fármaco,* o una *droga de abuso.* *Adicciones 2007*; 19 (3): 225- 238.

[2] Bordeaux B, Lieberman H. Benefits and risks of caffeine and caffeinated beverages. UpToDate. Literature review current through: Nov 2013. This topic last updated: oct 25, 2013. Accesed: Dic 28, 2013. Available from: http://www.uptodate.com/

[3] Kent A. Sepkowitz, MD. Energy Drinks and Caffeine-Related Adverse Effects. *JAMA*, 2013; 309(3): 243-244.

[4] Tavares C, Sakata K. Cafeína para el tratamieto del dolor. *Rev. Bras. Anestesiol.* 2012; 62: 3: 387-401.

[5] Calle S. *Determinación analítica de la cafeína en diferentes productos comerciales.* [Proyecto de fin de carrera]. Barcelona: Universitat Politècnica de Catalunya 2011.

[6] Kerrigan S, Lindsey T. *Fatal caffeine overdose: Two case reports. Forensic Science International 2005. 153,* 67-69.

[7] Essayan DM. Cyclic nucleotide phosphodiesterases. *J. Allergy Clin. Inmunol.* 2001, 108 (5): 671-680.

[8] Daly JW, Jacobson KA, Ukena D. Adenosine receptors: development of selective agonists and antagonists. *Prog. Clin. Biol. Res.* 1987, 230 (1): 41-63.

[9] Bennet AW, Bonnie BK. El mundo de la cafeína. Madrid 2013. *Editorial Fondo de Cultura Económica de España.* ISBN 978-6-07-160943-4. pp 225-238.

[10] Reissig CJ, Strain EC, Griffiths. Caffeinated energy drinks-A growing problem. *Drug and alcohol dependence* 2009, 99: 1-10.

[11] Torpy JM, Livingston EH. Energy Drinks. *JAMA* 2013, 309 (3): 297.

[12] Wolk BJ, Ganetsky M, Babuc KM. Toxicity of energy drinks. *Curr Opin Pediatr* 2012, 24: 243 – 251.

[13] Chin JM, Merves ML, Golberger BA, Sampson-Cone A, Cone EJ. Caffeine content of brewed teas. *J. Anal. Toxicol.* 2008, 32: 702-704.

[14] Vademécum Internacional Medicom. *Medimedia-Medicom*, SA, Madrid 2013.p 87-752.

[15] Underm BJ. Brunton LL, Lazo JS, Parker KL. Pharmacotherapy of asthma. Goodman & Gilman. *The Pharmacological Basis of Therapeutics.* 11th ed. New Cork: McGrawHill, 2006. p. 717-36.

[16] Childs E, de Wit H. Subjective, behavioral, and physiological effects of acute caffeine in light, nondependent caffeine users. *Psychopharmacol* 2006; 185: 514- 523.

[17] Ker K, Edwards PJ, Felix LM, et al. Caffeine for the prevention of injuries and errors in shift workers. *Cochrane Database Syst Rev* 2010, Issue 5. Art Nº: CD008508. DOI: 10.1002/14651858. CD008508.

[18] Sadock BJ, Sadock VA. Kaplan & Sadock. Sinopsis de Psiquiatría. 10ª Edición. *Editorial Lippincot* W&W, 2009. ISBN 978-84-96921-38-2.

[19] Sawynok J. Methylxanthines and pain. *Handb Exp. Pharmacol.* 2011, 200: 311-329.

[20] Grace Giardina E. *Cardiovascular effects of caffeine.* UpToDate. Literature review current through: Dec 2013. This topic last updated: sept, 2013. Accesed: Dic 28, 2013. Available from: http://www. uptodate.com/

[21] Mehta A, Jain AC, Mehta MC, Billie M. Caffeine and cardiac arrhythmias. An experimental study in dogs with review of literature. *Acta Cardiol* 1997; 52 (3): 273-283.

[22] Chelsky LB, Cutler JE, Griffith K, et al. Caffeine and ventricular arrhythmias. An electrophysiological approach. *JAMA* 1990; 264 (17): 2236-2240.

[23] Corti R, Binggeli C, Sudano I, et al. Coffee acutely increases sympathetic nerve activity and blood pressure independently of caffeine content: role of habitual versus nonhabitual drinking. *Circulation* 2002; 106: 2935-2940.

[24] Cornelis MC, El-Sohemy A, Kabagambe EK, Campos H. Coffee, CYP1A2 genotype, and risk of myocardial infarction. *JAMA* 2006; 295: 1135-1141.

[25] Schmidt B, Roberts RS, Davis P et al. Caffeine therapy for apnea of prematurity. *N. Engl. J. Med.* 2006; 354: 2112-2121.

[26] Golfrank LR, Hoffman RS, Nelso LS, Howland MA, Lewin NA, Flomenbaum NE. *Golfrank's Manual of Toxicologic Emergencies. Methylxanthines.* Eighth Edition. United States of America: Mc Graw Hill; 2007. p. 553-559.

[27] Daly JW. Caffeine analogs: biomedical impact. *Cell Mol. Life Sci.* 2007, 64: 2153-2169.

[28] Bara AI, Barley EA. Caffeine for asthma. *Cochrane Database Syst. Rev.* 2000;2: CD001112.

[29] Fisone G, Borgkvist A, Usiello A. Caffeine as a psychomotor stimulant: mechanism of action. *Cell Mol. Life Sci.* 2004; 61:857-872.

Caffeine 81

[30] Maughan RJ, Griffint J. Caffeine ingestion and fluid balance: a review. *The British Dietetic Association*, 2003. 16: 411-420.

[31] Ribeiro JA, Sebastião AM. Caffeine and adenosine. *J. Alzh Dis.* 2010, 20: S3-S15.

[32] Burke LM. Caffeine and sports performance. *Appl. Physiol. Nutr. Metab.* 2008; 33:1319-1334.

[33] Korpelainen R, Korpelainen J, Heikkinen J, et al. Lifestyle factors are associated with osteoporosis in lean women but not in normal and overweight women: a population-based cohort study of 1222 women. *Osteoporos Int.* 2003; 14:34-43.

[34] Laurence AS, Wight J, Forrest AR. Fatal theophylline poisoning with rhabdomyolysis. *Anaesthesia.* 1992; 47:82: 1365-2044.

[35] Tianying Wu, Walter C. Willett, Susan E. Hankinson, Edward Giovannucci. Caffeinated Coffee, Decaffeinated Coffee, and Caffeine in Relation to Plasma C-Peptide Levels, a Marker of Insulin Secretion, in U.S. Women. *Diabetes Care* 2005;28:1390-1406.

[36] Cote-Menendez M. Bebidas energizantes: ¿Hidratantes o estimulantes?. *Rev. Fac. Med.* 2011 Vol. 59 (3): 255-266.

[37] Cheung RJ Gupta EK, Ito MK. Acute Coffee Ingestion Does Not Affect LDL Cholesterol Level. *Ann. Pharmacother* 2005, 39: 1209-1213.

[38] Nisenblat V, Norman R J, Lockwood CJ, Barss VA. The effects of caffeine on reproductive outcomes in women. Literature review current through: Dec 2013. This topic last updated: sep 11, 2013. Avalaible on line in: www.uptodate.com Accesed september 2013.

[39] Hatch E, Lauren A, Mikkelsen EM, Christensen T, Riis AH, Sorensen HT, Rothmana KJ. Caffeinated Beverage and Soda Consumption and Time to Pregnancy. *Epidemiology* 2012; 23: 393– 401.

[40] Arria A, O´Brien MC. The "High" Risk of Energy Drinks. *JAMA* 2011, 305 (6): 600-601.

[41] Frost P, Vestergaard P. Caffeine and risk of atrial fibrillation or flutter: the Danish Diet, Cancer, and Health Study. *Am. J. Clin. Nutr.*, 2005. 81(3): 578-582.

[42] Cua WL, Pease JA, Stewart JT. A Case of Ventricular Tachycardia Related to Caffeine Pretreatment. *J. ECT* 2009; 25: 70-71.

[43] Artin B, Singh M, Richeh C, Jawad E, Arora R, Khosla S. Caffeine-Related Atrial Fibrillation. *American Journal of Therapeutics* 2010, 17:e169–e171.

[44] Townsend MK, Resnick NM, Grodstein F. Caffeine Intake and Risk of Urinary Incontinence Progression Among Women. *Obstet. Gynecol.* 2012;119:950–957.

[45] Jura YH, Townsedn MK, Curham GC, Resnick NM, Grodstein F. Caffeine intake, and the risk of stress, urgency and mixed urinary incontinence. *J. Urol.* 2011, 185(5): 1775-1780.

[46] Gleason JL, Richter HE, Redden DT, Goode PS, Burgio KL, Markland AD. Caffeine and urinary incontinence in US women. *Int. Urogynecol. J.* 2013, 24(2): 295-302.

[47] Nicole J. Davis, C.P.V., Theodore M. Johnson, and K.L.B. Patricia S. Goode, David T. Redden and Alayne D. Markland, Caffeine Intake and its Association with Urinary Incontinence in United States Men: Results from National Health and Nutrition Examination Surveys 2005–2006 and 2007–2008. *The Journal of Urology* 2012, 189: 2170-2174.

[48] Tsimihodimos V, Kakaldi V, Elisaf M. Cola-induced hypokalaemia: pathophysiological mechanisms and clinical implications. *Int. J. Clin. Pract.*, June 2009, 63 (6): 900–902.

[49] Rigato G, Blarasin L, Kette F. Severe Hypokalemia in 2 Young Bicycle Riders Due to Massive Caffeine Intake. *Clin. J. Sport Med.* 2010, 20:128–130.

[50] Babu KM, Zuckerman MD, Cherkes JK, Hack JB. First-Onset Seizure After Use of 5-hour ENERGY. *Pediatr Emer Care* 2011, 27: 539-540.

[51] Mortelmansa L, Van Looa M, De Cauwerb HG, Merlevedeb K. Seizures and hyponatremia after excessive intake of diet coke. *European Journal of Emergency Medicine* 2008, 15:51.

[52] Macleod MR. White PM. Not tonight, Darling, I might get a headache. *Stroke.* 2011, 42:1807-1808.

[53] Aurora RN, Crainiceaun C, Caffo B, Punjabi NM. Sleep-Disordered Breathing and Caffeine Consumption. Results of a Community-Based Study. *CHEST* 2012; 142(3):631–638.

[54] Kapur R, Smith M. Treatment of cardiovascular collapse from caffeine overdose with lidocaine, phenylephrine, and hemodialysis. *American Journal of Emergency Medicine* 2009, 27, 253.e3–253.e6.

[55] Yew D, Tarabar A. Caffeine toxicity. Updated: Sept 3, 2013. Available on line in: http://emedicine.medscape.com/article/821863-overview Accesed in september 2013.

[56] Fernández-Miret B, Castaño S, Maynar J, Iturbe M, Barrasa H, Corral E. Intoxicación aguda grave por cafeína. A propósito de 2 casos con 2 cursos diferentes. *Med. Intensiva.* 2013;37(6): 431—436.

Caffeine 83

[57] Lopez-Garcia E, Van Dam RM, Li TY, Rodríguez-Artalejo F, Hu FB. The Relationship of Coffee Consumption with Mortality. *Ann. Intern Med.* 2008,148: 904-914.

[58] Brice CF, Smith AP. Effects of caffeine on mood and performance: a study of realistic consumption. *Psychopharmacology* 2002, 164: 188-192.

[59] Kato E, Wellons M, Lipman TO, Lin FH. Benefits and risks of caffeine and caffeinated beverages. Literature review current through: Dec 2013. This topic last updated: oct 25, 2013. Avalaible on line in: www.uptodate.com Accessed september 2013.

[60] Shy BD, Portelli I, Nelson LS. Emergency medicine residents' use of psychostimulants and sedatives to aid in shift work. *American Journal of Emergency Medicine* 2011, 29: 1034–1036.

[61] Samuels CH. Jet Lag and Travel Fatigue: A Comprehensive Management Plan for Sport Medicine Physicians and High-Performance Support Teams. *Clin. J. Sport Med.* 2012, 22:268–273.

[62] Sökmen B, Armstrong LE, Kraemer WJ, Casa DJ, Dias JC, Judelson DA, Maresh CM. Caffeine use in sports: considerations for the athlete. *Journal of Strength and Conditioning Research* 2008, 22(3): 978–986.

[63] Caffeine-related disorders. In: American Psychiatric Association: *Diagnostic and Statistical Manual of Mental Disorders: DSM-IV*, Fourth Edition. Washington, DC, American Psychiatric Association, 1994. p. 212-5.

[64] Rihs M, Muller C, Bauman P. Caffeine consumption in hospitalized psychiatric patients. *Eur. Arch. Psychiatry Clin. Neurosci.* 1996, 246: 83-92.

[65] Ferre S. An update on the mechanisms of the psychoestimulant effects of caffeine. *J. Neurochem.* 2008, 105: 1067-1079.

[66] Fredholm BB, Bättig K, Holmen J, Nehlig A, Zvartau EE. Actions of caffeine in the brain with special reference to factors that contribute to its widespread use. *Pharmacol. Rev.* 1999, 51. 83-133.

[67] Fredholm BB, Chen JF, Cunha RA, Svenningsson P, Vaugeois JM. Adenosine and brain function. *Int. Rev. Neurobiol.* 2005, 63: 191-270.

[68] Lara DR. Caffeine, Mental Health, and Psychiatric Disorders. *J. Alzheimers Dis.* 2010, 20 Suppl 1: S239-248.

[69] Lader M, Bruce M. States of anxiety and their induction by drugs. *Br. J. Clin. Pharmacol.* 1986, 22(3): 251–261.

[70] Silverman K, GriffithsRR. Low-dose caffeine discrimination and self-reported mood effects in normal volunteers. *J. Exp. Anal. Behav.* 1992, 57(1): 91-107.

[71] Ogawa N, Ueki H. Secondary mania caused by caffeine. *Gen. Hosp. Psychiatry.* 2003, 25 (2): 138-139.

[72] Caykoylu A, Ekinci O, Kuloglu M. Improvement from treatment-resistant schizoaffective disorder, manic type after stopping heavy caffeine intake: a case report. *Prog. Neuropsychopharmacol. Biol. Psychiatry* 2008, 32: 1349-1350.

[73] Hedges DW, Woon FL, Hoopes SP. Caffeine-induced psychosis. *CNS Spectr.* 2009, 14: 127-129.

[74] Lucas PB, Pickar D, Kelsoe J, Rappaport M, Pato C, Hommer D. Effects of the acute administration of caffeine in patients with schizophrenia. *Biol. Psychiatry* 1990, 28: 35-40.

[75] Ramos JA, Collazos F, Casas M. Metilxantinas. In: Bobes J, Casas M, Gutierrez M, editores. Manual de evaluación y tratamiento de drogodependencias. Ars Medica 3 ed. Barcelona, 2003. p. 335-342.

[76] Pentel P. Toxicity of over-the-counter stimulants. *JAMA* 1984, 252: 1898-903.

[77] Strain EC, Mumford GH, Silverman K, Grifiths RR. Caffeine dependence síndrome: evidence from case histories and experimental evaluations. *JAMA* 1994, 272: 1043-8.

[78] Juliano LM, Griffiths RR. Caffeine. In: Lowinson JH, Ruiz P, Millman RB, Langrod JG, editors. *Substance Abuse. A Comprehensive Textbook.* Lippincott Williams & Wilkins, Philadelphia, 2005. p. 403-421.

[79] Moro MA, Lizasoain I, Ladero JM. Xantinas. In: Lorenzo P, Ladero JM, Leza JC, Lizasoain I. Drogodependencias. Panamericana 3 ed. Madrid 2009. p. 295-302.

[80] Griffiths RR, Woodson PP. Caffeine physical dependence: a review of human and laboratory animal studies. *Psychopharmacology* (Berl). 1988, 94: 437-51.

[81] Sadock B. Sadock V. Kaplan & Sadock's. Synopsis of Psychiatry Caffeine related disorders. Behavioral Sciences / Clinical Psychiatry. Lippincott Williams & Wilkins 10 ed. Philadelphia, 2009. p. 412-416.

[82] Silverman K, Evans SM, Strain EC, Griffiths R. Withdrawal syndrome after the double blind cessation of caffeine consumption. *N. Engl. J. Med.* 1992, 327: 1109-1114.

[83] Hughes JR, Oliveto AH, Bickel WK, Helzer JE. Indications of caffeine dependence in a population based sample. En: Harris LS, editor.

Problems of drug dependence, 1992, NIDA Research Monographs Series. Washington: Governments Printing Office, 1993. p. 194-198.

[84] Juliano LM, Griffiths RR. A critical review of caffeine withdrawal: empirical validation of symptoms and signs, incidence, severity, and associated features. *Psychopharmacology* (Berl). 2004, 176: 1-29.

[85] Henderson-Smart DJ, Steer PA. *Methylxanthine treatment for apnea in preterm infants.* Cochrane Database of Systematic Reviews 2001, Issue 3. Art. No.: CD000140. DOI: 10.1002/14651858. CD000140.

[86] Dukhovny D, Lorch SA, Schmidt B, Doyle LW, Kok JH, Roberts RS, Kamholz KL, Na Wang MA, Mao W, Zupancic JA. Economic evaluation of caffeine for apnea of prematurity. *Pediatrics,* 2011, 127(1): e146-55.

[87] Dasheiff R. Modafinil is not the new caffeine. *Neurology* 2010, 75: 1764-1765.

[88] Wright K, Badia P, Myers B, Plenzler S. Combination of bright light and caffeine as a countermeasure for impaired alertness and performance during extended sleep deprivation. *J. Sleep Res.* 1997, 6(1): 26-35.

[89] Wyatt JK, Cajoche C, Ritz-De Cecco A, Czeisler CA, Dijk DJ. Low-dose repeated caffeine administration for circadian-phase-dependent performance degradation during extended wakefulness. *Sleep* 2004, 27(3): 374-81.

[90] Schweitzer PK, Randazzo AC, Stone K, Erman M, Walsh JK. Laboratory and field studies of naps and caffeine as practical countermeasures for sleep-wake problems associated with night work. *Sleep* 2006, 29 (1): 39-50.

[91] Mednick SC, Cai DJ, Kanady J, Drummond S. Comparing the benefits of caffeine, naps and placebo on verbal, motor and perceptual memory. *Behav. Brain Res.* 2008, 193(1): 79-86.

[92] Ferrauti A, Weber K, Struder HK. Metabolic and ergogenic effects of carbohydrate and caffeine beverages in tennis. *J. Sports Med. Phys. Fitness* 1997, 37(4): p. 258-66.

[93] Davis JM, Zhao Z, Stock HS, Mehl KA, Buggy J, Hand GA. Central nervous system effects of caffeine and adenosine on fatigue. *Am. J. Physiol. Regul. Integr. Comp. Physiol.*, 2003, 284(2): R399-404.

[94] Hernán MA, Takkouche B, Camaño-Isorna F, Gestal-Otero JJ. A meta-analysis of coffee drinking, cigarette smoking, and the risk of Parkinson's disease. *Ann. Neurol.* 2002, 52 (3):276-284.

[95] Postuma, R.B., Caffeine for treatment of Parkinson disease. *Neurology* 2012, 79: 651-658.

[96] Barranco Quintana JL. Alzheimer`s disease and coffee: a quantitative review. *Neurol. Res.* 2007; 29:91.

[97] Yoovathaworn, K.C., K. Sriwatanakul, and A. Thithapandha, Influence of caffeine on aspirin pharmacokinetics. *Eur. J. Drug Metab. Pharmacokinet.* 1986, 11(1): 71-76.

[98] Iqbal N, Ahmad B, Janbaz KH, Gilani AH, Niazi SK. The effect of caffeine on the pharmacokinetics of acetaminophen in man. *Biopharm. Drug Dispos* 1995, 16(6): 481-487.

[99] Ward N, Whitney C, Avery D, Dunner D. The analgesic effects of caffeine in headache. *Pain* 1991, 44(2): 151-155.

[100] Camann WR, Murray RS, Mushlin PS, Lambert DH. Effects of oral caffeine on postdural puncture headache. A double-blind, placebo-controlled trial. *Anesth Analg* 1990, 70(2): 181-184.

[101] Benton R, Hunter RA, Are There Pharmacologic Agents That Safely and Effectively Treat Post–Lumbar Puncture Headache? *Annals of Emergency Medicine* 2013, 61 (1): 84-85.

[102] Mercadante S, Serretta R, Casuccio A. Effects of caffeine as an adjuvant to morphine in advanced cancer patients. A randomized, double-blind, placebo-controlled, crossover study. *J. Pain Symptom Manage* 2001, 21(5): 369-372.

[103] Shapiro R. Caffeine and headaches. *Neurol. Sci.* 2007. 28 Suppl 2: S179-83.

[104] Renner E, Wietholtz H, Huguenin, Arnaud PM, Preisig R. Caffeine: a model compound for measuring liver function. *Hepatology* 1984, 4(1): 38-46.

[105] Wang, T, Kleber G, Stellaard F, Paumgartner G. Caffeine elimination: a test of liver function. *Klin. Wochenschr* 1985, 63(21): 1124-1128.

[106] Desmond PV,Patwardhan RV, Johnson RF, Schenker S. Impaired elimination of caffeine in cirrhosis. *Dig. Dis. Sci.* 1980, 25(3): 193-197.

[107] Perlik F, Pucelikova T, Slanar O. Use of the paraxanthine/caffeine ratio in the saliva of patients with liver cirrhosis. *Cas Lek Cesk* 2001,140(2): 51-53.

[108] Cheng W, Murphy T, Smith MT, Cooksley GE, Halliday JW, Powel LW. Dose-dependent pharmacokinetics of caffeine in humans: Relevance as a test of quantitative liver function. *Clin. Phamacol. Ther.* 1990, 47(4): 516-524.

[109] Mostofsky E, Rice MS, Levitan EB, Mittleman MA. Habitual coffee consumption and risk of heart failure: a dose-response meta-analysis. *Circ. Heart Fail* 2012. 5(4): 401-5.

[110] Van Dam RM, Hu FB. Coffe consumption adn risk of type 2 diabetes. *JAMA* 2005, 294: 97-104.

[111] Huxley R, Lee CMY, Barzi F Timmermeister L, Czernichow S, Perkovic V, Grobbee DE, Batty D, Woodward M. Coffe, decaffeinated coffe, and tea consumption in relation to incident type 2 diabetes mellitus. *Arch. Intern Med.* 2009, 169(22): 2053-2063.

[112] Leitzmann MF, Stampfer MJ, Willet WC, Spiegelman D, Colditz GA, Giovannucci EL. Coffee intake is associated with lower risk of symptomatic gallstone disease in women. *Gastroenterology* 2002, 123(6): 1823-1830.

[113] Leitzmann MF, Willett W, Rim EB, Stampfer MJ, Spiegelman D, Colditz GA, Giovannucci E. A prospective study of coffee consumption and the risk of symptomatic gallstone disease in men. *JAMA* 1999, 281: 2106-2112.

[114] Walcher T, Haenle MM, Mason RA, Koenig W, Imhof A, Kratzer W for the EMIL Study Group. The effect of alcohol, tobacco and caffeine consumption and vegetarian diet on gallstone prevalence. *Eur. J. Gastroenterol. Hepatol.* 2010, 22: 1345-1351.

[115] Carrillo JA, Benitez J. Clinically significant pharmacokinetic interactions between dietary caffeine and medications. *Clin. Pharmacokinet.* 2000, 39 (2): 127-153.

In: Caffeine	ISBN: 978-1-63117-777-4
Editor: Aimée S. Tolley	© 2014 Nova Science Publishers, Inc.

Chapter 4

CAFFEINE MODULATION OF ALCOHOL INTAKE: IMPACT ON ITS PSYCHOMOTOR EFFECTS AND WITHDRAWAL

M. Correa[1,2,], N. San Miguel[1], L. López-Cruz[1], P. Bayarri[1] and J. D. Salamone[2]*

[1]Àrea de Psicobiologia, Campus de Riu Sec, Universitat Jaume I,
Castelló, Spain
[2]Department of Psychology, University of Connecticut, Storrs, CT, US

ABSTRACT

The impact of caffeine on ethanol consumption and abuse has become a topic of great interest due to the rise in popularity of "energy drinks". Energy drinks have many different components, although the main active ingredient is caffeine. These drinks are frequently taken in combination with alcohol under the belief that caffeine can offset some of the intoxicating effects of ethanol. However, scientific research has not universally supported the idea that caffeine can reduce the effects of ethanol in humans or in rodents, and the mechanisms mediating caffeine-ethanol interactions are not well understood. Caffeine and ethanol have a common biological substrate; both act on neurochemical processes

---

[*] Corresponding author: Mercè Correa, Ph.D. Area de Psicobiologia, Universitat Jaume I, Campus Riu Sec, 12071 Castelló, Spain. Tel: +34-964-729841. Fax: +34-964-729267. E-mail address: correa@psb.uji.es.

related to the neuromodulator adenosine. Caffeine acts as a non-selective adenosine A_1 and A_{2A} receptor antagonist, while ethanol has been demonstrated to increase the basal adenosinergic tone via multiple mechanisms. Since adenosine transmission modulates multiple behavioral processes, the interaction of both drugs can regulate a wide range of behavioral effects, which can have an impact on alcohol consumption and the development of alcohol addiction. In the present review we discuss epidemiological studies and laboratory animal work that have assessed the impact of caffeine on alcohol consumption. In addition, we evaluate how caffeine can also affect the consumption of other drugs of abuse. Finally we present data on human and animal studies analyzing the impact of caffeine on alcohol withdrawal, and psychomotor performance.

CAFFEINE AS A "NEW" DRUG OF ABUSE

Caffeine intake, even in excess, is well accepted socially because methylxanthines have activating and attention-preserving properties that can help productivity and enhance performance. However, interest in caffeine abuse has grown ever since the introduction to the market of the so-called "energy drinks". Although energy drinks contain several components with clear psychoactive effects, such as taurine or glucose, recent studies show that caffeine is the active ingredient responsible for the behavioral and cognitive effects associated with these beverages (Giles et al., 2012). In general, energy drinks contain caffeine in quite high concentrations. A cup of coffee contains about 100 mg of caffeine and a can of a traditional cola drink contains around 35 mg of caffeine. However, although the caffeine content of energy drinks varies considerably, the concentration of caffeine can be much higher than coffee or most sodas; it ranges from as low as 50 mg to ten times more, up to 500 mg of caffeine per unit (Reissig et al., 2009).

The aggressive marketing of energy drinks targets young consumers, with advertising emphasizing that these drinks induce states of arousal and psychological 'highs'. In fact, some slogans of well known energy drinks emphasize the idea that these drinks procure energy, increase endurance, and produce a sense of invincibility. It is quite common to see campaigns that offer free samples on college campuses and venues where this segment of the population concentrates. In the United States 34% of young people aged between 18 and 24 are consumers of energy drinks (O'Brien et al. 2008; Wells et al., 2013), and among college students percentages of consumption rise to 60% (Price et al., 2010). In addition, these drinks are often consumed in combination with other substances that have abuse potential (Morelli and Simola, 2011).

CAFFEINE: SYNERGY WITH OTHER DRUGS OF ABUSE

Caffeine has a facilitating effect on the self-administration of other drugs. Energy drink users are significantly more likely than nonusers to initiate nonmedical use of prescription stimulants and prescription analgesics (Arria et al., 2010). Several reports indicate that cigarette smokers consume more caffeine than nonsmokers (Parsons and Neims, 1978; Swanson et al., 1994), an effect that may be partially due to increased caffeine metabolism among cigarette smokers (Parsons and Neims, 1978). However, in a laboratory context acute high doses of caffeine given to smokers did not increase cigarette smoking, probably because they report increases in anxiety and dysphoric somatic effects (Chait and Griffiths, 1983). Results obtained in animals show that squirrel monkeys that received intramuscular injections of caffeine increased lever-pressing for nicotine (Prada and Goldberg, 1985; Yasar et al., 1997) and in rats, adding caffeine to the drinking water also increased intravenous nicotine self-administration (Shoaib et al., 1999).

Similar experimental results have been observed for cocaine. Caffeine administered in the food to rhesus monkeys produced a modest increase in self-administration of smoked cocaine (Comer and Carroll, 1996). In rats, it has been demonstrated that intraperitoneal (IP) injections of caffeine potentiated intravenous self-administration of cocaine (Horger et al., 1991; Schenk et al., 1994), and reinstated cocaine self-administration after the animal had stopped seeking for the drug (Schenk and Partridge, 1999).

The interaction of caffeine with opiates presents a different picture; in humans there seems to be little correlation between heroin abuse and caffeine consumption (Kozlowski et al., 1993). Similarly in animals, it has been demonstrated that both, acute and chronic caffeine intake, decreased morphine self-administration in rats, possible due to an increased in anxiety (Sudakov et al., 2002).

However, high doses of caffeine induced withdrawal signs in morphine-dependent monkeys (Aceto et al., 1978), and mice (Ahlijanian and Takemori 1985; 1986), as well as rats (Khalili et al., 2001), and also increased the naloxone-precipitated withdrawal effect (Capasso and Gallo, 2009).

In contrast, the severity of alcoholism was directly related to various measures of caffeinated beverage use (Kozlowski et al., 1993). Among all drugs of abuse studied, the one that has been demonstrated to be coadministered most frequently with caffeine or energy drinks is alcohol. Thus, this chapter will focus on the interaction between caffeine and alcohol.

EFFECT OF CAFFEINE ON ALCOHOL CONSUMPTION: EPIDEMIOLOGICAL STUDIES

Although the sporadic consumption of energy drinks, caffeinated sodas or coffees typically is not a problem in itself, combined with alcohol consumption can have many added risks. The combined intake of alcohol and energy drinks is a relatively new phenomenon that is increasing in frequency. Within the last 3 years there has been a proliferation of epidemiological studies assessing the incidence of combined consumption of energy drinks and alcohol, especially among teenagers and young adults from many different countries. Typically, combined consumption of these two drugs occurs in young social drinkers on a night-out who are motivated to drink alcohol heavily and to become intoxicated. For instance, around 50-65% of college students report consuming energy drinks to stay awake and study longer hours, but they also report that the main reason to use energy drinks is to be able to last longer when consuming alcohol at parties (Malinauskas et al., 2007; Oteri et al., 2007). Moreover, the combined use of energy drinks and alcohol in young adults that are not college students in nightclubs (17.1%) is also lower than that generally found in college student samples (Wells et al., 2013).

The reasons for combining caffeine with ethanol may stem from the popular belief that caffeine can antagonize the intoxicating effects of alcohol (Hasenfratz et al., 1993). It has been described that these energy drinks reduce sleepiness, increase energy and also the perceived sense of wellbeing, when combined with alcohol (Malinauskas et al., 2007; O'Brien et al., 2008). This very popular idea may be a factor contributing to the positive correlation between consumption of caffeine and that of ethanol (Marczinski et al., 2012). People who use energy drinks consume alcohol more frequently than people who do not. Around half of the college students who consume alcohol regularly report that they do mixed it with energy drinks (O'Brien et al., 2008; Malinauskas et al., 2007; Oteri et al., 2007; Attila and Çakir, 2011), and, among those students who drink alcohol, the amount consumed is greater if they do it with energy drinks (Price et al., 2010; Patrick and Maggs 2013). High frequency users of energy drinks consume alcohol more frequently and in higher quantities, increasing the risk of alcohol overdose (Patrick and Maggs, 2013). The consumption of alcohol mixed with energy drinks in students is strongly associated with high-risk drinking behavior, including increased binge drinking, more frequent episodes of weekly drunkenness, and elevated blood alcohol content (O'Brien et al., 2008; Patrick and Maggs, 2013). High frequency users of energy drinks and ethanol were also twice as likely to meet Diagnostic and Statistical Manual of Mental Disorders 4th edition (DSM-IV) criteria for alcohol dependence, compared with low frequency users (Arria et al., 2011; American Psychiatric Association, 2000).

Furthermore, it appears that energy drinks change the palatability of alcohol when used as a mixer; the high glucose content of these drinks makes beverages with high alcohol content easier to drink, especially for naïve and early consumers with little experience in the consumption of alcohol. Compared to low-frequency energy drink users, high-frequency users were reported to be significantly more likely to have gotten intoxicated at an early age (Arria et al., 2011). Thus, one of the clear risks of the combined consumption is that young people seem to end up consuming more alcohol and doing so earlier in life.

EFFECT OF CAFFEINE ON ALCOHOL CONSUMPTION: LABORATORY STUDIES

A limited number of studies employing experimental animal models have been performed to elucidate the impact of caffeine on alcohol consumption. Studies in rodents have shown a complex relationship between caffeine administration and ethanol intake. Studies of chronic administration show that caffeine administered in the diet facilitates voluntary ethanol drinking in rats in a free access two-bottle paradigm (Gilbert, 1976; 1979), and removal of caffeine from the diet restored alcohol consumption to baseline levels. However, slow-release caffeine pellets failed to alter ethanol intake in a similar paradigm (Potthoff et al., 1983). The presence of caffeine in alcoholic solutions did not increase ethanol consumption in rats exposed to a free-choice procedure (Carvalho et al., 2012). Interestingly, it did prevent the alcohol deprivation effect, blocking the typical increase of ethanol intake after an abstinent period (Carvalho et al., 2012). Caffeine administered acutely did not produce a consistent pattern of effects either; a low dose of caffeine (5.0 mg/kg, intraperitoneally, IP) promoted ethanol drinking in rats using a limited-access two-bottle choice paradigm (Kunin et al., 2000). However, a high acute dose of caffeine (50.0 mg/kg, IP) decreased ethanol as well as food intake in rats (Dietze and Kulkosky, 1991).

Caffeine has been shown to indirectly modulate the activity of many neurotransmitters and neuromodulators, among which the most direct action is on adenosine receptors (Fredholm et al., 1999). Caffeine acts as a nonselective antagonist for A_1 and A_{2A} receptor subtypes in the central nervous system (CNS). (Fredholm et al., 1999, 2001; Cauli and Morelli, 2005; Ferré et al., 2008) Adenosine produces hypnotic and anxiolytic effects as well as a reduction of locomotion (Deckert, 1998; Correa and Font, 2008), while caffeine blocks adenosine's sedative, anxiolytic and sleep-inducing effects. Ethanol increases adenosine levels by potentiating adenosine release (Clark and Dar, 1989; Fredholm and Wallman-Johansson, 1996) and by decreasing adenosine uptake (Diamond and Gordon, 1997; Ruby et al., 2010). Secondarily, ethanol increases adenosine levels because acetate generated by ethanol metabolism promotes adenosine synthesis (Carmichael et al., 1991; Pardo et al., 2013a). Furthermore, adenosine seems to mediate alcohol-induced motor incoordination, hypnotic effects, and anxiolysis (Dar et al., 1994; Israel et al., 1994; Correa and Font, 2008; Batista et al., 2005). Thus, caffeine and ethanol seem to have opposite actions on the same neuromodulator. Alterations in adenosinergic signaling mediate many of the effects of acute ethanol administration, particularly with regard to motor function and sedation (Israel et al., 1994; Pardo et al., 2013a).

Research on the role of adenosine receptor subtypes in ethanol intake has mainly focused on A_{2A} receptors. Ethanol intake increased in A_{2A} KO mice compared to their WT counterparts in a free choice task (Naassila et al., 2002). Similarly, acute and subchronic administration of A_{2A} receptor antagonists increased ethanol intake in alcohol-preferring rats in a free choice paradigm (Micioni Di Bonaventura et al., 2012). In operant chambers, in which animals have to exert effort to have access to ethanol (e.g. lever pressing), the pattern of effects produced by different A_{2A} receptor antagonists was more complex. While some increased, others reduced the number of ethanol-reinforced responses and ethanol consumption (Adams et al., 2008; Thorsell et al., 2007). No effect was observed with an adenosine A_1 antagonist (Arolfo et al., 2004).

Taken together, it appears that the results from animal studies so far are not conclusive. The specific effects of adenosine antagonism on ethanol self-administration may depend on factors such as food restriction, sex, ethanol-intake or reinforcement paradigms, or other factors. For instance, it has been suggested that the suppressive effects of caffeine on ethanol intake seen in some studies could be due to the use of high toxic doses of caffeine (Itsvan and Matarazzo, 1984).

EFFECT OF CAFFEINE ON ALCOHOL WITHDRAWAL

Withdrawal is a defining characteristic of drug dependence and is often characterized by impaired physiological function and enhanced negative affect, symptoms strongly associated with relapse (Breese et al., 2005). Some symptoms of ethanol withdrawal appear starting as soon as 12 hrs after the time when ethanol levels in blood are no longer detectable. For instance, acute withdrawal appears several hours after a high dose of ethanol has been administered, and produces a mild set of symptoms (i.e., hangover). Beliefs about the effects of mixing caffeine and alcohol on hangover or sleep may play a role in the motivation to consume mixtures of the two substances. However, recent studies show that this mixture does not affect amount of sleep or sleep latency, hangover, or sleepiness the morning after drinking to intoxication levels (Penning et al., 2011; Rohsenow et al., 2014).

Among other effects, acute and chronic withdrawal from ethanol typically includes anxiety symptoms (Breese et al., 2005). In addition, high doses of caffeine have been demonstrated to induce anxiety in humans and rodents (For a review see Correa and Font 2008). Recently, in humans it has been reported that consumption of energy drinks (100 mL/day) also was significantly associated with anxiety (but not depression or stress) in young adult males (Trapp et al., 2013). Thus, the popular belief that a cup of strong coffee can antagonize some of the symptoms of ethanol-withdrawal, seems to be counterintuitive in the case of anxiety. Chronic ethanol exposure and withdrawal affect mainly A_1 receptor density in rodents (for a review see Butler and Prendergast, 2012) and although the impact of selective adenosine antagonists on anxiety induced by ethanol withdrawal has been investigated in a handful of studies (for a recent review see López-Cruz et al., 2013), leading to the conclusion that A_1 agonists attenuate and A_1 antagonists exacerbate the anxiogenic effect of ethanol withdrawal (Butler and Prendergast, 2012), there are no data so far directly assessing the impact of caffeine on ethanol withdrawal.

In mice, we recently demonstrated that an acute dose of caffeine (25.0 or 50.0 mg/kg) induces anxiogenic responses in an elevated plus maze (López-Cruz et al., 2011). Using the same testing parameters, we evaluated the impact of previous exposure to caffeine in mice that, after drinking ethanol for a long period of time, went through repeated episodes of withdrawal. Adult C57BL/6JRccHsd male mice (Harlan Labs. Spain) had 24 hours access to two different bottles of tap water (control group) or one of tap water and the other of ethanol 10% w/v (withdrawal group) during 10 weeks. In the last 6 weeks of this period, both groups received a dose of caffeine (0, 2.5, 5.0, 10.0, 20.0 and 40.0 mg/kg, IP) once a week. Every mouse received all doses in a random order. After these 10 weeks the ethanol solution was removed for 4 days, after which it was reintroduced for another 4 days. This cycle of removal and reintroduction of ethanol in the withdrawal group was repeated 3 times. Both groups had continuous access to water. Four days after the last ethanol removal, animals in control and experimental groups received either saline or a dose of 40.0 mg/kg of caffeine, and were evaluated in the elevated plus maze (see figures 1A-D) for measures of anxiety (latency to enter an open arm, time spent in the open arms, and ratio between entries in the open arms and total entries), and a measure of locomotion (total number of entries). The two-way factorial ANOVA (intake solution x dose of caffeine) for the four dependent variables lead to the following results: latency (no effect of the intake solution, caffeine dose $[F_{(1,39)}=3.82, p<0.05]$, and interaction $[F_{(1,39)}=12.53, p<0.01]$), time in open arms (no effect of caffeine dose, intake factor $[F_{(1,39)}=8.23, p<0.001]$, and interaction $[F_{(1,39)}=6.49, p<0.01]$), ratio (caffeine dose $[F_{(1,39)}=4.03, p<0.05]$, intake factor $[F_{(1,39)}=8.95, p<0.01]$, and interaction $[F_{(1,39)}=9.93, p<0.01]$) and for total arm entries (no effect of caffeine dose, the intake factor $[F_{(1,39)}=8.95, p<0.01]$, and interaction $[F_{(1,39)}=12.53, p<0.01]$). Because all the interactions were significant LSD post hoc test were conducted to compare groups (results are shown in the graphs).

Thus, the water (control) group did not show an anxiogenic response to a challenge of 40.0 mg/kg of caffeine, as do animals exposed for the first time to this drug at high doses (López-Cruz et al., 2011). This result seems to be caused by the repeated administration of caffeine once a week for 5 weeks at doses ranging from 2.5-40.0 mg/kg that all the mice in the present experiment had received. In fact, 40.0 mg/kg caffeine induced an anxiolytic response in the control mice, as well as increased locomotion.

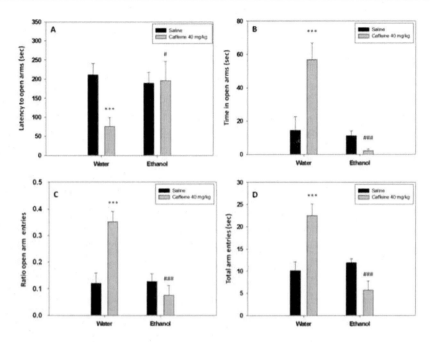

Figure 1. Effect of acute administration of caffeine (0 or 40 mg/kg, IP) in mice pre-exposed to water or to several cycles of ethanol withdrawal on the elevated PM (N=11-13 per group). All mice had also previous repeated experience with caffeine (2.5 - 40 mg/kg, IP). Data are expressed as mean (± SEM) of A) latency (sec) to enter an open arm, B) time (sec) spent in the open arms, C) ratio of open arm entries, and D) total arm entries during 5 minutes. ***$p<0.001$ significant differences between doses of caffeine in the same intake group. #$p<0.05$, ###$p<0.001$ significant differences between the same dose of caffeine in different intake groups.

It seems then that repeated caffeine administration at a younger age inoculates an animal from the anxiogenic impact of acute effects of caffeine later in life. However, the group that had consumed ethanol did not show the anxiolytic effect of this dose of caffeine. The two groups of saline treated animals were no different from each other. Thus, ethanol pre-exposed animals did not show enhanced anxiety as compared to water-exposed mice 4 days after ethanol removal, but this previous treatment was able to block the anxiolytic effect of previous experience with caffeine.

Although there are no other animal studies focusing on the impact of caffeine on anxiety induced by ethanol withdrawal, our results generally agree with a study in male rats chronically exposed during adolescence to caffeine and ethanol in the drinking water (Hughes et al., 2011). After interruption of the treatment, animals were tested in adulthood for anxiety in an open field and in a dark-light box. The group that during adolescence consumed both caffeine plus ethanol showed a significantly higher anxiolytic behavior compared to animals exposed only to ethanol (Hughes et al., 2011).

CAFFEINE AND ALCOHOL INTERACTION: SUBJECTIVE, COGNITIVE AND PSYCHOMOTOR EFFECTS

In addition to the impact of caffeine on alcohol consumption and abuse, public health concerns also arise from reports of increased risk of alcohol-related negative consequences (Patrick and Maggs, 2013; O'Brien et al., 2008; Arria et al., 2011; Berger et al., 2011; Howland et al., 2011). A significant number of consumers of caffeine-alcohol mixes use them before or during work, which increases the frequency of accidents in manual occupations (Cheng et al., 2012). Moreover, the consumption of alcohol mixed with energy drinks has been strongly associated with a higher prevalence of serious alcohol-related consequences; including being sufficiently sick or injured as a result of drinking to seek medical attention, being taken advantage of sexually, having unprotected sex, riding with a drunken driver, or driving while intoxicated (O'Brien et al., 2008; Berger et al., 2013). Drinkers who reported mixing alcohol with energy drinks had a threefold higher risk of being legally intoxicated and a fourfold increase in the probability of reporting the intention to drive a motor vehicle, compared with drinkers who reported consuming alcohol alone (Thombs et al., 2010). It is this last harmful consequence that appears to have a higher impact among young people (Fudin and Nicastro, 1988).

The combination of high doses of caffeine and alcohol induces the so called 'wide-awake drunk' (Attwood, 2012). This can lead to a person underestimating the level of intoxication, which can lead to drinking for longer periods of time, increasing the risk of reaching higher blood alcohol levels that exceed the legal limits for driving. Risks associated with alcohol consumption increase after consuming 5 or more drinks for men and 4 for women in a short period of time (O'Brien et al., 2008). This pattern is considered as hazardous or "binge drinking", and is very typical among young alcohol consumers (NIAAA 2011). In the U.S., 51 % of drivers aged 18-24 years who died in traffic accidents in recent years had alcohol levels above the permissible blood levels, and although there is not a relation between blood alcohol levels and subjective intoxication among energy drink consumers, higher blood levels were associated with a greater number of negative consequences (Patrick and Maggs, 2013).

The ability to evaluate our own and others' level of alcohol intoxication is a very important component of risk assessment (O'Brien et al., 2008), and combining alcohol with energy drinks can mask the signs of alcohol intoxication. Energy drinks with high caffeine content have been demonstrated to improve subjective measures of mood, concentration, and feelings of alertness (Alford et al., 2001; Seidl et al., 2000), and the majority of consumers of energy drinks mixed with alcohol do so to reduce the sedative effects and lack of coordination that alcohol produces at high doses, and also to increase the stimulant effects that alcohol has at low doses.

However, the sedative and incoordination effects that can be an important part of the intoxication feeling after consuming ethanol, do not seem to be clearly improved by caffeine. Some studies in humans tested under laboratory conditions show that participants report feeling less intoxicated or impaired when caffeine and alcohol are co-administered (Ferreira et al., 2006; Marczinski and Fillmore, 2006). However, there are also data showing that alcohol-related impairment of cognitive and motor function seems to remain largely unaffected by consuming caffeine (Weldy, 2010; Ulbrich et al., 2013). In this regard, several studies show no significant changes in subjective feelings of depression, anxiety, drunkenness or subjective intoxication, subjective impairment, and sedation (Arria et al., 2011; Azcona et al., 1995; Peacock et al., 2013).

It has been suggested that with the addition of caffeine to alcohol, the qualitative change in intoxication is due mainly to an increase in self-reported stimulation, although not necessarily a quantitative reduction in intoxication per se (Attwood et al., 2011). Moderate increases in subjective stimulation ratings are observed after consuming both substances (Peacock et al., 2013), and laboratory studies in humans suggest that there appear to be mild stimulant-like effects on performance of objective tasks such as reaction time, digit symbol substitution, rapid information processing tasks, and memory recall (Azcona et al., 1995; Drake et al., 2003; Hasenfratz et al., 1993; Howland et al., 2010, Mackay et al., 2002). Caffeine attenuates ethanol-induced changes in psychological parameters such as information processing, memory, and psychomotor performance (Ferré and O'Brien, 2011). In contrast, in a classic study, the combination of alcohol plus caffeine produced no impact on reaction time compared to the alcohol alone group (Azcona et al., 1995). Also, in inhibitory control tasks such as go-no-go, or stop-signal, reports show mixed findings (Ferré and O'Brien, 2011). Thus, caffeine improves alcohol-related detriment on some tasks, while having no effect, or even worsening performance, on others (Fillmore and Vogel-Sprott, 1999; Marczinski and Fillmore, 2003; Attwood et al., 2011).

It is possible that these discrepant findings are a result of the use of different methodologies. There seems to be a lack of consensus on the required dose of caffeine to reduce the psychomotor depressant effects of alcohol in humans. For example, a concentration of caffeine of 80.0 mg given in an energy drink may not be sufficient to antagonize the effects of medium doses of alcohol (0.6 and 1.0 g / kg) (Ferreira et al., 2004). Although this combination of doses reduced the subjective feeling of intoxication characterized as decrease in headache, reduced feelings of fatigue, less dizziness, fewer problems when walking, or less dry mouth (Ferreira et al., 2004; 2006), in a test of visual motor coordination physiological parameters and biochemical and behavioral measures assessed objectively, such as alcohol concentration in exhaled air or performance and reaction time, were not changed (Ferreira et al., 2004; 2006). Again, it appears that the subjective feeling of alcohol intoxication is reduced by caffeine, but not the intoxication itself (Riesselmann et al., 1996).

In another study, a higher concentration of caffeine (400 mg) plus a low dose of alcohol (0.6 g/kg) improved psychomotor performance in relation to individuals who consumed only alcohol. However, no improvement on parameters such as the ability to drive a car in a simulator was observed (Liguori and Robinson, 2001). Results indicate that legally intoxicated individuals cannot antagonize alcohol-induced, driving-related decrements with caffeine prior to driving an automobile (Fudin and Nicastro, 1988), thought to be the major behavior for which caffeine is used in attempts to antagonize alcohol-induced decrements, confirming the idea that consumers of energy drinks and alcohol may have a reduced subjective sense of intoxication (Riesselmann et al., 1996), thereby increasing the likelihood of accidents when combining both substances.

Animal studies, show that both drugs are able to stimulate locomotor activity in rodents at some dose (Arizzi-LaFrance et al., 2006; Correa et al., 2003; 2009; López-Cruz et al., 2011), and low doses of caffeine can increase motor stimulant properties of moderate doses of alcohol, (Waldeck, 1974; Kuribara et al., 1992; López-Cruz et al., 2012). However, high doses of caffeine, such as those contained in energy drinks, have been shown to increase the motor incoordination produced by high doses of alcohol (López-Cruz et al., 2012). Pilcher (1911) concluded years ago that "when small doses of caffeine and alcohol are combined, the result is generally a qualitative algebraic summation of both actions, i.e. each drug produces, qualitatively, its ordinary effects. However, when large doses of the two drugs are combined, the effects of the stimulant drug tend to be reversed, resulting in a greater suppression than the suppressant drug alone" (Pilcher, 1911).

CONCLUSION

Caffeine has been shown to have beneficial and therapeutic effects in motor performance. For example, low doses of caffeine and its metabolite theophylline have been shown to improve motor symptoms in humans and in animal models of Parkinson disease (Fredholm et al., 1999; Salamone et al., 2008; Pardo et al., 2013b). In addition, low doses of caffeine plus ethanol, equivalent to no more than 2 to 3 cups of strong coffee and 1 cocktail, reduce stroke damage in experimental models, and this effect is now in clinical evaluation for treatment of ischemic stroke, with promising effects (Martin-Schild et al., 2009).

In spite of this beneficial effects of low doses of both substances, concentrations of caffeine in energy drinks are so high than if a person consumes several of these energy drinks on a single episode (i.e., a binge over a few hours), he or she can end up self-administering a high dose of caffeine that is unlikely to have therapeutic effects. The European Commission and the American Food and Drug Administration (FDA) report that, in humans, when blood alcohol concentrations are low, low doses of caffeine can produce a "modest" effect on motor parameters. But this does not occur when doses and concentrations of both substances are high (European Commission Health & Consumer Protection Directorate- General, 2007), as is the case during many instances of recreational drug use.

Young people who consume energy drinks also drink alcohol more frequently and in higher quantities. Alcohol facilitates exposure to anxiogenic or risky situations, produces psychomotor disinhibition, and promotes impulsive behavior. In young people, perceived risk associated with alcohol consumption is determined by variables such as perceived control over the situation. A factor that increases this sense of control is the use of substances to "reduce the effects of alcohol." Combining alcohol with energy drinks can lead to a sense of control over the intoxicating effects of alcohol by virtue of masking signs of alcohol intoxication, which then results in greater levels of alcohol intake, dehydration, more severe and prolonged hangovers, and ultimately, alcohol poisoning.

Numerous brands of alcohol/caffeine combination drinks have been produced. Positive effects of caffeine/alcohol combination drinks are readily and aggressively relayed in marketing campaigns. But negative effects, if relayed at all, appear as 'small print' on labels that consumers often fail to read. Current European legislation (European Directive 2002/67/EC on the labeling of food containing caffeine) rules that beverages containing up to 150 mg/l must be marked as 'high caffeine content' and that this statement should be in the same field of vision as the product name. In 2010, the US Food and Drug Administration issued warnings to several manufacturers of combination drinks identifying caffeine as an 'unsafe food additive' mixed with alcohol, and stated that their sale violated federal law. There are also restrictions on the production and sale of caffeinated alcohol beverages in some countries, including Canada, where caffeine can only be mixed with alcohol if it comes from a natural source (e.g. guarana), and Mexico, where caffeinated alcohol beverage sales are prohibited in bar rooms and night clubs. In the UK, alcohol-related harm and binge drinking are high on the political agenda, and there have been calls for legal restrictions on the amount of caffeine that can be added to alcohol products.

Thus, different countries have already adopted strategies to avoid mixing alcohol with energy drinks. A number of countries have a requirement on manufacturers to label drinks, indicating the possibility that the mixture affects the perceived levels of intoxication. However, the debate over caffeinated alcohol beverages is somewhat undermined by the fact that caffeinated energy drinks are widely available. Although they have been banned in various countries in the past (e.g. France, Denmark, Norway), many of these bans have since been revoked. And individuals are still free to mix their own caffeine/alcohol beverages. In conclusion, public health concern over caffeinated alcohol drinks is justified, although the nature of the caffeine/alcohol relationship is yet to be fully elucidated.

ACKNOWLEDGMENTS

This work was supported by a grant to Mercè Correa from Plan Nacional de Drogas (2010/024), Spain, and to John Salamone from the National Institute of Mental Health (MH078023). Laura López-Cruz was supported by a personal grant awarded by FPU (AP2010-3793) Ministerio de Educación, Spain, and Noemí San Miguel was supported by Predoc-UJI/ 2012/28.

REFERENCES

Aceto, M.D., Carchman, R.A., Harris, L.S. & Flora, R.E. (1978). Caffeine elicited withdrawal signs in morphine-dependent rhesus monkeys. *Eur. J. Pharmacol.,* 50(3), 203-7.

Adams, C.L., Cowen, M.S., Short, J.L., & Lawrence, A.J. (2008). Combined antagonism of glutamate mGlu5 and adenosine A2A receptors interact to regulate alcohol-seeking in rats. *Int J Neuropsychopharmacol.,* 11(2), 229-41.

Ahlijanian, M.K. & Takemori, A.E. (1985). Effects of (-)-N6-(R-phenylisopropyl)-adenosine (PIA) and caffeine on nociception and morphine-induced analgesia, tolerance and dependence in mice. *Eur. J. Pharmacol.,* 112(2), 171-9.

Ahlijanian, M.K. & Takemori, A.E. (1986). The effect of chronic administration of caffeine on morphine-induced analgesia, tolerance and dependence in mice. *Eur. J. Pharmacol.,* 120(1), 25-32.

Alford, C., Cox, H. & Wescott, R.(2001).The effects of red bull energy drink on human performance and mood. *Amino Acids,* 21(2), 139-50.

American Psychiatric Association. (2000). *Diagnostic and Statistical Manual of Mental Disorders* (Revised 4th ed.). Washington, DC.

Arizzi-LaFrance, M.N., Correa, M., Aragon, C.M.G. & Salamone, J.D. (2006). Motor stimulant effects of ethanol injected into the substantia nigra pars reticulata: importance of catalase-mediated metabolism and the role of acetaldehyde. *Neuropsychopharmacology,* 31(5), 997-1008.

Arolfo, M.P., Yao, L., Gordon, A.S., Diamond, I. & Janak, P.H. (2004). Ethanol operant self-administration in rats is regulated by adenosine A2 receptors. *Alcohol Clin Exp Res.* 8(9), 1308-16.

Arria, A.M., Caldeira, K.M., Kasperski, S.J., O'Grady, K.E., Vincent, K.B., Griffiths, R.R. et al. (2010). Increased alcohol consumption, nonmedical prescription drug use, and illicit drug use are associated with energy drink consumption among college students. *J. Addict. Med.,* 4(2), 74-80.

Arria, A.M., Caldeira, K.M., Kasperski, S.J., Vincent, K.B., Griffiths, R.R. & O'Grady, K.E. (2011). Energy drink consumption and increased risk for alcohol dependence. *Alcohol. Clin. Exp. Res.,* 35(2), 365-75.

Attila, S. & Çakir, B. (2011). Energy-drink consumption in college students and associated factors. *Nutrition,* 27(3), 316-22.

Attwood, A.S., Rogers, P.J., Ataya, A.F., Adams, S. & Munafò, M.R. (2011). Effects of caffeine on alcohol-related changes in behavioural control and perceived intoxication in light caffeine consumers. *Psychopharmacology* (Berl), 221(4), 551-60.

Attwood, A.S. (2012). Caffeinated alcohol beverages: a public health concern. *Alcohol Alcohol*, 47(4), 370-1.

Azcona, O., Barbanoj, M.J., Torrent, J. & Jané, F. (1995). Evaluation of the central effects of alcohol and caffeine interaction. *Br. J. Clin. Pharmacol.*, 40, 393-400.

Batista, L.C., Prediger, R.D., Morato, G.S. & Takahashi, R.N. (2005). Blockade of adenosine and dopamine receptors inhibits the development of rapid tolerance to ethanol in mice. *Psychopharmacology*, 181(4), 714-21.

Berger, L.K., Fendrich, M., Chen, H.Y., Arria, A.M. & Cisler, R.A. (2011). Sociodemographic correlates of energy drink consumption with and without alcohol: results of a community survey. *Addict Behav.*, 36(5), 516-9.

Berger, L., Fendrich, M. & Fuhrmann, D. (2013). Alcohol mixed with energy drinks: are there associated negative consequences beyond hazardous drinking in college students?. *Addict. Behav.*, 38(9), 2428-32.

Breese, G.R. Overstreet, D.H. & Knapp, D.J. (2005). Conceptual framework for the etiology of alcoholism: a "kindling"/stress hypothesis. *Psychopharmacology*, 178(4), 367-80.

Butler, T.R. & Prendergast, M.A. (2012). Neuroadaptations in adenosine receptor signaling following long-term ethanol exposure and withdrawal. *Alcohol Clin. Exp. Res.*, 36(1), 4-13.

Capasso, A. & Gallo, C. (2009). Functional interaction between purinergic system and opioid withdrawal: in vitro evidence. *Curr. Drug Saf.*, 4(2), 97-102.

Carmichael, F.J., Israel, Y., Crawford, M. et al. (1991). Central nervous system effects of acetate: contribution to the central effects of ethanol. *J. Pharmacol. Exp. Ther.*, 259(1), 403-8.

Carvalho, C.R., Cruz, J.S. & Takahashi, R.N. (2012). Prolonged exposure to caffeinated alcoholic solutions prevents the alcohol deprivation effect in rats. *J. Caffeine Res.*, 2, 83-9.

Cauli, O. & Morelli, M. (2005). Caffeine and the dopaminergic system. *Behav. Pharmacol.*, 16, 63-77.

Chait, L.D. & Griffiths, R.R. (1983). Effects of caffeine on cigarette smoking and subjective response. *Clin. Pharmacol. Ther.*, 34(5), 612-22.

Cheng, W., Cheng, Y., Huang, M. & Chen, C.J. (2012). Alcohol dependence, consumption of alcoholic energy drinks and associated work characteristics in the Taiwan working population. *Alcohol Alcohol,* 47, 372-9.

Clark, M. & Dar, M.S. (1989). Effect of acute ethanol on release of endogenous adenosine from rat cerebellar synaptosomes. *J. Neurochem.,* 52(6), 1859-65.

Comer, S.D. & Carroll, M.E. (1996). Oral caffeine pretreatment produced modest increases in smoked cocaine self-administration in rhesus monkeys. *Psychopharmacology,* 126(4), 281-5.

Correa, M., Arizzi, M.N., Betz, A., Mingote, S. & Salamone, J.D. (2003). Locomotor stimulant effects of intraventricular injections of low doses of ethanol in rats: acute and repeated administration. *Psycopharmacology.* 170 (4), 368-75.

Correa, M. & Font, L. (2008). Is there a major role of A2A adenosine receptor in anxiety? *Front. Biosci.,* 13, 4058-70.

Correa, M., Viaggi, C., Escrig, M.A., Pascual, M., Guerri, C., Vaglini, F. et al. (2009). Ethanol intake and ethanol-induced locomotion and locomotor sensitization in Cyp2e1 knockout mice. *Pharmacogenet. Genomics,* 19(3), 217-25.

Dar, M.S., Bowman, E.R. & Li, C. (1994). Intracerebellar nicotinic-cholinergic participation in the cerebellar adenosinergic modulation of ethanol-induced motor incoordination in mice. *Brain Res.,* 644(1), 117-27.

Deckert, J. (1998). The adenosine A(2A) receptor knockout mouse: a model for anxiety? *Int. J. Neuropsychopharmacol.,* 1(2), 187-90.

Diamond, I. & Gordon, A.S. (1977). Cellular and molecular neuroscience of alcoholism. *Physiol. Rev.,* 77(1), 1-20.

Dietze, M.A. & Kulkosky, P.J. (1991). Effects of caffeine and bombesin on ethanol and food intake. *Life Sci.,* 48(19),1837-44.

Drake, C.L., Roehrs, T., Turner, L., Scofield, H.M. & Roth, T. (2003). Caffeine reversal of ethanol effects on the multiple sleep latency test, memory, and psychomotor performance. *Neuropsychopharmacology,* 28(2), 371-8.

European Commission Health & Consumer Protection Directorate-General. (2007). *Opinion of the Scientific Committee on Food on Additional information on "energy" drinks.* http://ec.europa.eu/food/fs/sc/scf/out169_en.pdf. Accessed Aug 9.

Ferré, S., Ciruela, F., Borycz, J. et al. (2008). Adenosine A1-A2A receptor heteromers: new targets for caffeine in the brain. *Front. Biosci.,* 13, 2391-9.

Ferré, S. & O'Brien, M.C. (2011). Alcohol and caffeine: the perfect storm. *J. Caffeine Res.*, 1, 153-62.

Ferreira, S.E., de Mello, M.T., Rossi, M.V. & Souza-Formigoni, M.L. (2004). Does an energy drink modify the effects of alcohol on a maximal effort test? *Alcohol Clin. Exp. Res.*, 28(9), 1408-12.

Ferreira, S.E., de Mello, M.T., Pompéia, S. & de Souza-Formigoni, M.L. (2006). Effects of energy drink ingestion on alcohol intoxication. *Alcohol Clin. Exp. Res.*, 30, 598-605.

Fillmore, M.T. & Vogel-Sprott, M. (1999). An alcohol model of impaired inhibitory control and its treatment in humans. *Exp. Clin. Psychopharmacol.*, 7(1), 49-55.

Fredholm, B.B. & Wallman-Johansson, A. (1996). Effects of ethanol and acetate on adenosine production in rat hippocampal slices. *Pharmacol. Toxicol.*, 79,120-3.

Fredholm, B.B., Bättig, K., Holmén, J. et al. (1999). Actions of caffeine in the brain with special reference to factors that contribute to its widespread use. *Pharmacol. Rev.*, 51(1), 83-133.

Fredholm, B.B., Ijzermanm A.P., Jacobson, K.A., Klotz, K.N. & Linden, J. (2001). International Union of Pharmacology: XXV. Nomenclature and classification of adenosine receptors. *Pharmacol. Rev.*, 53(4), 527-52.

Fudin, R. & Nicastro, R. (1988). Can caffeine antagonize alcohol-induced performance decrements in humans?. *Percept. Motor Skills*, 67(2), 375-91.

Gilbert, RM. (1976). Dietary caffeine and EtOH consumption by rats. *J. Stud. Alcohol*, 37(1), 11-8.

Gilbert, R.M. (1979). Augmentation of EtOH-consumption by caffeine in malnourished rats. *J. Stud. Alcohol*, 40(1), 19-27.

Giles, G.E., Mahoney, C.R., Brunyé, T.T., Gardony, A.L., Taylor, H.A. & Kanarek, R.B. (2012). Differential cognitive effects of energy drink ingredients: Caffeine, taurine, and glucose. *Pharmacol. Biochem. Behav.*, 102, 569-77.

Hasenfratz, M., Bunge, A., Dal Prá, G. & Bättig K. (1993). Antagonistic effects of caffeine and alcohol on mental performance parameters. *Pharmacol. Biochem. Behav.*, 46(2), 463-5.

Horger, B.A., Wellman, P.J., Morien, A., Davies, B.T. & Schenk, S. (1991). Caffeine exposure sensitizes rats to the reinforcing effects of cocaine. *Neuroreport*, 2(1), 53-6.

Howland, J., Rohsenow, D.J., Arnedt, J.T., Bliss, C.A., Hunt, S.K., Calise, T.V. et al. (2010). The acute effects of caffeinated versus non-caffeinated alcoholic beverage on driving performance and attention/reaction time. *Addiction*, 106(2), 335-41.

Howland, J., Rohsenow, D.J., Calise, T.V., Mackillop, J. & Metrik, J. (2011). Caffeinated alcoholic beverages: an emerging public health problem. *Am. J. Prev. Med.*, 40(2), 268-71.

Hughes, R.N. (2011). Adult anxiety-related behavior of rats following consumption during late adolescence of alcohol alone and in combination with caffeine. *Alcohol*, 45(4), 365-72.

Israel, Y, Orrego, H. & Carmichael, F.J. (1994). Acetate-mediated effects of ethanol. *Alcohol Clin. Exp. Res.*, 18(1), 144-8.

Itsvan, J. & Matarazzo, J.D. (1984). Tobacco, alcohol, and caffeine use: a review of their interrelationships. *Psychol. Bull.*, 95, 301-26.

Kalodner, C.R., Delucia, J.L. & Ursprung, A.W. (1989). An examination of the tension reduction hypothesis: the relationship between anxiety and alcohol in college students. *Addict. Behav.*, 14(6), 649-54.

Khalili, M., Semnanian, S. & Fathollahi, Y. (2001). Caffeine increases paragigantocellularis neuronal firing rate and induces withdrawal signs in morphine-dependent rats. *Eur. J. Pharmacol.*, 412(3), 239-45.

Kozlowski, L.T., Henningfield, J.E., Keenan, R.M., Lei, H., Leigh, G., Jelinek, L.C. et al. (1993). Patterns of alcohol, cigarette, and caffeine and other drug use in two drug abusing populations. *J. Subst. Abuse Treat.*, 10(2), 171-9.

Kunin, D., Gaskin, S., Rogan, F., Smith, B.R. & Amit, Z. (2000). Caffeine promotes ethanol drinking in rats. Examination using a limited-access free choice paradigm. *Alcohol*, 21(3), 271-7.

Kuribara, H., Asahi, T. & Tadokoro, S. (1992). Ethanol enhances, but diazepam and pentobarbital reduce the ambulation-increasing effect of caffeine in mice. *Arukoru Kenkyuto Yakubutsu Ison*, 27(5), 528-39.

Liguori, A. & Robinson, J.H. (2001). Caffeine antagonism of alcohol-induced driving impairment. *Drug Alcohol Depend.*, 63(2), 123-9.

López-Cruz, L., Pardo, M., San Miguel, N., Salamone, J.D. & Correa, M. (2012). *Impact of high doses of caffeine on acute and sensitized motor activity induced by ethanol in mice.* Pp: 594. http://w3.kenes-group.com/congress/fens2012/pdf/FENS-FORUM-2012-Programme.pdf.

López-Cruz, L., Salamone, J.D. & Correa, M. (2013). The impact of caffeine on the behavioral effects of ethanol related to abuse and addiction: a review of animal studies. *J. Caffeine Res.*, 3(1), 9-21.

López-Cruz, L., Pardo, M., Dosda, A., Salamone, J.D. & Correa, M. (2011). Comparison between high doses of caffeine and theophylline on motor and anxiogenic effects in CD1 mice: studies of acute and chronic administration. *Behav. Pharmacol.* 22, 71-2.

Mackay, M., Tiplady, B. & Scholey, A.B. (2002). Interactions between alcohol and caffeine in relation to psychomotor speed and accuracy. *Hum. Psychopharmacol.,* 17(3), 151-6.

Malinauskas, B.M., Aeby, V.G., Overton, R.F., Carpenter-Aeby, T. & Barber-Heidal, K. (2007). A survey of energy drink consumption patterns among college Students. *Nutr. J.,* 6, 35.

Marczinski, C.A. & Fillmore, M.T. (2003). Dissociative antagonistic effects of caffeine on alcohol-induced impairment of behavioral control. *Exp. Clin. Psychopharmacol.* 11, 228-36.

Marczinski, C.A. & Fillmore, M.T. (2006). Clubgoers and their trendy cocktails: implications of mixing caffeine into alcohol on information processing and subjective reports of intoxication. *Exp. Clin. Psychopharmacol.,* 14(4), 450-8.

Marczinski, C.A., Fillmore, M.T., Henges, M.A., Ramsey, M.A. & Young, C.R. (2012). Effects of energy drinks mixed with alcohol on information processing, motor coordination and subjective reports of intoxication. *Exp Clin Psychopharmacol.,* 20(2),129-38.

Martin-Schild, S., Hallevi, H., Shaltoni, H., Barreto, A.D., Gonzales, N.R., Aronowski, J., Savitz, S.I. & Grotta, J.C. (2008). Combined neuroprotective modalities coupled with thrombolysis in acute ischemic stroke: a pilot study of caffeinol and mild hypothermia. *J. Stroke Cerebrovasc. Dis.,* 18(2), 86-96.

Micioni Di Bonaventura, M.V., Cifani, C., Lambertucci, C., Volpini, R., Cristalli, G., Froldi, R. & Massi, M. (2012). Effects of A2A adenosine receptor blockade or stimulation on alcohol intake in alcohol-preferring rats. *Psychopharmacology.* 219(4), 945-57.

Morelli, M. & Simola, N. (2011). Methylxanthines and drug dependence: a focus on interactions with substances of abuse. In: *Methylxanthines.* B.B. Fredholm (Ed). Heidelberg, Germany: Springer; 2011: pp. 484-501.

Naassila, M., Ledent, C. & Daoust, M. (2002). Low ethanol sensitivity and increased ethanol consumption in mice lacking adenosine A2A receptors. *J Neurosci.* 22(23), 10487-93.

O'Brien, M.C., McCoy, T.P., Rhodes, S.D., Wagoner, A. & Wolfson, M. (2008). Caffeinated cocktails: energy drink consumption, high-risk drinking, and alcohol-related consequences among college students. *Acad. Emerg. Med.,* 15(5), 453-60.

Oteri, A., Salvo, F., Caputi, A.P. & Calapai, G. (2007). Intake of energy drinks in association with alcoholic beverages in a cohort of students of the School of Medicine of the University of Messina. *Alcohol Clin. Exp. Re.,* 31(10), 1677-80.

Pardo, M., Betz, A.J., San Miguel, N., López-Cruz, L., Salamone, J.D. & Correa, M. (2013a). Acetate as an active metabolite of ethanol: studies of locomotion, loss of righting reflex, and anxiety in rodents. *Front. Behav. Neurosci.,* 7, 81.

Pardo, M., López-Cruz, L., Valverde, O., Ledent, C., Baqi, Y., Müller, C.E., Salamone, J.D. & Correa, M. (2013b). Effect of subtype-selective adenosine receptor antagonists on basal or haloperidol-regulated striatal function: studies of exploratory locomotion and c-Fos immunoreactivity in outbred and A2AR KO mice. *Behav. Brain Res.,* 247, 217-26.

Parsons, W.D. & Neims, A.H. (1978). Effect of smoking on caffeine clearance. *Clin. Pharmacol. Ther.,* 24(1), 40-5.

Patrick, M.E. & Maggs, J.L. (2013). Energy Drinks and Alcohol: Links to Alcohol Behaviors and Consequences Across 56 Days. *J. Adolesc. Health.* pii: S1054-139X(13)00511-9. doi: 10.1016/j.jadohealth.2013.09.013.

Peacock, A., Bruno, R., Martin, F.H. & Carr, A. (2013). The impact of alcohol and energy drink consumption on intoxication and risk-taking behavior. *Alcohol Clin. Exp. Res.,* 37(7), 1234-42.

Penning, R., de Haan, L. & Verster. J.C. (2011). Caffeinated Drinks, Alcohol Consumption, and Hangover Severity. *Open Neuropsychopharmacol. J.,* 4, 36-9.

Pilcher, J.D. (1911). Alcohol and caffeine: a study of antagonism and synergism. *J. Pharmacol. Exp. Ther.,* 8, 267-98.

Prada, J.A. & Goldberg, S.R., (1985). Effects of caffeine or nicotine pretreatments on nicotine self-administration by the squirrel monkey. *Psychopharmacologist* 27, 226.

Price, S.R., Hilchey, C.A., Darredeau, C., Fulton, H.G. & Barrett, S.P. (2010). Energy drink co-administration is associated with increased reported alcohol ingestion. *Drug Alcohol Rev.,* 29(3), 331-3.

Potthoff, A.D., Ellison, G., & Nelson, L. (1983). Ethanol intake increases during continuous administration of amphetamine and nicotine, but not several other drugs. *Pharmacol. Biochem. Behav.,* 18(4), 489-93.

Reissig, C.J., Strain, E.C. & Griffiths, R.R. (2009). Caffeinated Energy Drinks -- A Growing Problem. *Drug Alcohol Depend.,* 99(1-3), 1-10.

Riesselmann, B., Rosenbaum, F. & Schneider, V. (1996). Alcohol and energy drink—can combined consumption of both beverages modify auto- mobile driving fitness? *Blutalkohol*, 33, 201-8.

Rohsenow, D.J., Howland, J., Alvarez, L., Nelson, K., Langlois, B., Verster, J.C. et al. (2014). Effects of caffeinated vs. non-caffeinated alcoholic beverage on next-day hangover incidence and severity, perceived sleep quality, and alertness. *Addict. Behav.*, 39(1), 329-32.

Ruby, C.L., Adams, C.A., Knight, E.J., Nam, H.W. & Choi, D.S. (2010). An essential role for adenosine signaling in alcohol abuse. *Curr. Drug Abuse Rev.*, 3, 163-74.

Salamone, J.D., Ishiwari, K., Betz, A., Farrar, A.M., Mingote, S.M., Font, L. & Correa, M. (2008). Dopamine/adenosine interactions related to locomotion and tremor in animal models: possible relevance to parkinsonism. *Parkinson. Rel. Dis.*, 14 (2), S130-4.

Schenk, S., Valadez, A., Horger, B.A., Snow, S. & Wellman, P.J. (1994). Interactions between caffeine and cocaine in tests of self-administration. *Behav. Pharmacol.*, 5(2), 153-8.

Schenk, S. & Partridge, B. (1999). Cocaine-seeking produced by experimenter-administered drug injections: dose-effect relationships in rats. *Psychopharmacology* (Berl), 147(3), 285-90.

Seidl, R., Peyrl, A., Nicham, R. & Hauser, E. (2000). A taurine and caffeine-containing drink stimulates cognitive performance and well-being. *Amino Acids,* 19(3-4), 635-42.

Shoaib, M., Swanner, L.S., Yasar S. & Golberg, S.R. (1999). Chronic caffeine exposure potentiates nicotine self-administration in rats. *Psychopharmacology* (Berl), 142(4), 327-33.

Sudakov, S.K., Papazov, I.P., Lyupina, Y.V., Medvedeva, O.F., Figurina, I.V. & Rusakova, I.V. (2002). Effects of acute and chronic caffeine intake on intravenous self-administration of morphine in two rat strains. *Bull. Exp. Biol. Med.*, 134(4), 400-2.

Swanson, J.A., Lee, J.W. & Hopp, J.W. (1994). Caffeine and nicotine: a review of their joint use and possible interactive effects in tobacco withdrawal. *Addict. Behav.*, 19(3), 229-56.

Thombs, D.L., O'Mara, R.J., Tsukamoto, M., Rossheim, M.E., Weiler, R.M., Merves, M.L. et al. (2010). Event-level analyses of energy drink consumption and alcohol intoxication in bar patrons. *Addict. Behav.*, 35(4), 325-30.

Thorsell, A., Johnson, J. & Heilig, M. (2007). Effect of the adenosine A2a receptor antagonist 3,7-dimethyl-propargylxanthine on anxiety-like and depression-like behavior and alcohol consumption in Wistar Rats. *Alcohol Clin Exp Res.* 31(8), 1302-7.

Trapp, G.S, Allen, K., O'Sullivan, T.A., Robinson, M., Jacoby, P. & Oddy, W.H. (2013). Energy drink consumption is associated with anxiety in australian young adult males. *Depress. Anxiety.* doi: 10.1002/da.22175.

Ulbrich, A., Hemberger, S.H., Loidl, A., Dufek, S., Pablik, E., Fodor, S., Herle, M. & Aufricht, C. (2013). Effects of alcohol mixed with energy drink and alcohol alone on subjective intoxication. *Amino Acids*, 45(6), 1385-93.

Waldeck, B. (1974). Ethanol and caffeine: a complex interaction with respect to locomotor activity and central catecholamines. *Psychopharmacologia,* 36(3), 209-20.

Weldy, D.L. (2010). Risks of alcoholic energy drinks for youth. *J. Am. Board Fam. Med.,* 23(4), 555-8.

Wells, B.E., Kelly, B.C., Pawson, M., Leclair, A., Parsons, J.T. & Golub, S.A. (2013). Correlates of Concurrent Energy Drink and Alcohol Use among Socially Active Adults. *Am. J. Drug Alcohol Abuse*, 39(1), 8-15.

Yasar, S., Shoaib, M., Gasior, M., Jaszyna, M. & Goldberg, S.R. (1997). Facilitation of IV nicotine self-administration in squirrel monkeys by caffeine. *J. Psychopharmacol.* 11, A14.

In: Caffeine
Editor: Aimée S. Tolley

ISBN: 978-1-63117-777-4
© 2014 Nova Science Publishers, Inc.

Chapter 5

REGULATION MECHANISM OF CAFFEINE ON GLUCOSE TRANSPORT AND UPSTREAM SIGNALING PATHWAYS IN SKELETAL MUSCLE

Tatsuro Egawa[1,2,3,]*, Satoshi Tsuda[1,3], Taku Hamada[4], Katsumasa Goto[2] and Tatsuya Hayashi[1]

[1]Laboratory of Sports and Exercise Medicine,
Graduate School of Human and Environmental Studies,
Kyoto University, Kyoto, Japan
[2]Department of Physiology, Graduate School of Health Sciences,
Toyohashi SOZO University, Aichi, Japan
[3]Japan Society for the Promotion of Science,
Tokyo, Japan
[4]Laboratory of Exercise Physiology and Biochemistry,
Graduate School of Sport and Exercise Sciences,
Osaka University of Health and Sport Sciences (OUHS),
Osaka, Japan

ABSTRACT

Skeletal muscle is the major organ playing an important role in whole-body glucose metabolism. Caffeine (1,3,7-trimethylxanthine) has

---

* Phone, Fax: +81-50-2017-2283; E-mail: tatsuro.egawa@gmail.com.

been implicated in the regulation of skeletal muscle glucose metabolism, including insulin-dependent and -independent glucose transport. However, the precise mechanism of how caffeine modulates these phenomena has not been firmly established. In this review, we provide our recent experimental evidence linking caffeine to glucose transport and upstream signaling pathways in skeletal muscle.

The initial part of this chapter introduced the effect of caffeine on insulin-dependent signaling pathways of glucose transport in skeletal muscle.

Incubation of isolated muscle with caffeine suppressed insulin-dependent tyrosine phosphorylation of insulin receptor substrate (IRS)-1. This response was accompanied with inhibition of insulin-dependent signaling pathways; phosphorylation of phosphatidylinositol-3 kinase and Akt, and with inhibition of insulin-dependent glucose transport. In addition, caffeine enhanced phosphorylation of IRS-1 on the inhibitory site Ser^{307} and inhibitor-κB kinase (IKK). Suppression of the IKK/IRS-1 Ser^{307} cascade reduced the caffeine-mediated downregulation of IRS-1 tyrosine phosphorylation and insulin-dependent glucose transport. On the other hand, Ca^{2+} release inhibitor, dantrolene did not rescue the downregulations while suppressing 5'AMP-activated protein kinase (AMPK)/IRS-1 Ser^{789} cascade.

Intravenous injection of caffeine at a physiological dose (5 mg/kg) in rats inhibited the insulin-dependent IRS-1 tyrosine phosphorylation and Akt phosphorylation in skeletal muscle. The findings indicate that caffeine inhibits insulin-dependent glucose transport through IRS-1 dysfunction, IKK/IRS-1 Ser^{307}-dependently and Ca^{2+}- and AMPK-independently, in skeletal muscle.

The second part of this chapter introduced how caffeine acts on AMPK and which α isoform of AMPK (AMPKα1 and AMPKα2) is predominantly activated by caffeine in skeletal muscle. Incubation of rat skeletal muscles with caffeine at high doses (3 mM) resulted in cellular energy deprivation and activation of both AMPKα1 and AMPKα2, and Ca^{2+}/calmodulin-dependent protein kinase (CaMK) II. Caffeine stimulation at low dose (1 mM) did not cause energy deprivation and activation of AMPKα2 or CaMKII, but did activate AMPKα1. Intravenous injection of caffeine (5 mg/kg) in rat preferentially activated AMPKα1 in epitrochlearis muscle.

The findings indicate that caffeine activates AMPK and CaMKII in skeletal muscle through either an energy-dependent or -independent pathway, and AMPKα1 plays a pivotal role in insulin-independent glucose transport in physiological conditions.

The findings of these investigations provide valuable information about the regulation mechanism underlying the caffeine-induced metabolic changes that occur in skeletal muscle.

INTRODUCTION

Type 2 diabetes mellitus (T2DM) is one of the most rapidly increasing chronic diseases in the world [1, 2]. An estimated 285 million people worldwide are affected by T2DM, a number that is expected to reach 439 million by 2030 [2, 3]. T2DM is associated with microvascular and macrovascular diseases affecting several organs, including skeletal muscle, liver, heart, brain, and kidneys, and will become a serious burden on society in the near future [4]. Therefore, we should be aware of our health problems and work on diabetes prevention. In this context, it was recently noted that chronic treatment with phytochemicals, including caffeine, have antidiabetic effects.

A number of epidemiological studies have shown that long-term consumption of caffeinated beverages such as coffee (reviewed in [5]) and green tea [6] is associated with reducing a risk of T2DM. Caffeine (1,3,7-trimethylxanthine) is abundantly contained in coffee and green tea, so it is considered that caffeine is an active ingredient for prevention of T2DM. It has been reported that caffeine possibly reduces the risk of T2DM through enhanced β-cell functions [7], promotes weight loss [8], increases blood adiponectin levels [9], reduces inflammatory cytokines in the blood [10], reduces the adipose tissue inflammatory adipocytokines and in the hepatic genes relating to fatty acid synthesis [11], and abolishes superoxide production and enhances central insulin signaling [12]. In contrast, there are several reports indicating caffeine-induced whole-body glucose intolerance and insulin resistance [13-19]. Thus, whether caffeine has beneficial effects on glucose metabolism is not well-defined. In this chapter, we introduce our recent research about the effect of caffeine on glucose transport, a rate-limiting step for glucose utilization under physiological conditions and upstream signaling events, with a focus on insulin-dependent and insulin-independent signaling pathways in skeletal muscle.

Important Role of Skeletal Muscle Glucose Transport in Preventing T2DM

Skeletal muscle is the principal site of glucose metabolism in the body. Insulin and exercise (muscle contraction) are major physiological stimuli to glucose transport in skeletal muscle [20]. Under insulin-stimulated conditions, more than 80% of blood glucose is disposed in skeletal muscle i.e. insulin-dependent glucose transport [21]. Therefore, a defect of insulin action in skeletal muscle has major consequences on whole-body glucose homeostasis. On the other hand, exercise leads to the acute hypoglycemic effect, and this phenomenon is considered to be induced by an insulin-like effect that increases the glucose transport into contracting skeletal muscle i.e. insulin-independent glucose transport. Importantly, the contraction-mediated mechanism for controlling glucose transport remains intact in T2DM [22]. Thus, the insulin-independent mechanism underlying the exercise-induced upregulation of glucose transport in skeletal muscle helps to improve glycemic control in T2DM and may prevent non-diabetic people from developing glucose intolerance.

CAFFEINE-INDUCED INHIBITION OF INSULIN-DEPENDENT GLUCOSE TRANSPORT PATHWAY

Insulin-Dependent Glucose Transport in Skeletal Muscle

Glucose transport occurs by facilitated diffusion via glucose transporter 4 (GLUT4), the predominant glucose transporter isoform present in skeletal muscle. Both insulin and exercise increase skeletal muscle glucose transport through the translocation of GLUT4 from an intracellular location to the plasma membrane and T-tubules [23] (Figure 1).

The regulation of insulin-dependent signaling events of glucose transport in skeletal muscle are initiated from insulin binding to the extracellular α-subunit of the insulin receptor (IR), and thereby inducing rapid phosphorylation of the receptor (auto-phosphorylation) and insulin receptor substrate (IRS)-1 on tyrosine residues. Tyrosine phosphorylation of IRS-1 by the IR allows the binding and activation of class IA phosphatidylinositol 3-kinase (PI3K). This leads to the generation of the critical second messenger PI-3,4,5-triphosphate, which in turn triggers the activation of Akt [23]. Eventually, Akt substrate of 160 kDa (AS160) and TBC1D1, members of the Rab-GTPase family of proteins, regulate GLUT4 translocation [24].

Reduced tyrosine phosphorylation of IRS-1 and PI3K activation in animal models of insulin resistance and also in T2DM patients are linked to impaired glucose transport [25]. In addition, reduction of the IRS-1 protein level and its tyrosine phosphorylation are seen in 30% of subjects at high risk of T2DM [25, 26].

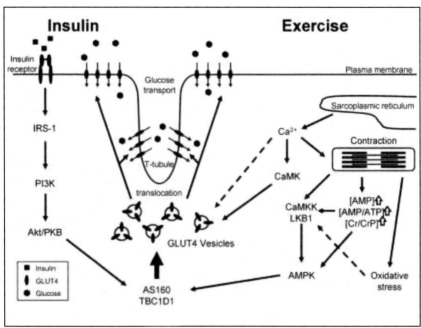

Adapted from Egawa et al. [101] with permission by the publisher.

Figure 1. Mechanisms of stimulating glucose transport by insulin and exercise (contraction).

Serine phosphorylation of IRS-1 seems to be attributed to impairment of tyrosine phosphorylation of IRS-1, thereby leading to an impairment of the insulin signaling cascade [27-30]. In fact, it was reported that serine phosphorylation of IRS-1 was elevated in the insulin-resistant state in human and rodent skeletal muscles [31, 32]. Thus, maintaining an insulin signaling cascade by a normal activation of IRS-1 plays an important role in prevention of T2DM.

Caffeine and Insulin Signaling Pathway in Skeletal Muscle

There are a number of reports demonstrating that caffeine administration acutely deteriorates whole-body insulin sensitivity in humans [13, 14, 16, 19, 33, 34]. In particular, it is speculated that caffeine-mediated insulin resistance occurs in skeletal muscle, judging that caffeine ingestion reduced insulin-stimulated glucose disposal during a hyperinsulinemic clamp [13, 14, 16]. However, the precise mechanism of caffeine-induced insulin resistance in skeletal muscle remains unclear. Recently, we demonstrated that caffeine-induce skeletal muscle insulin resistance is caused by IRS-1 dysfunction [35]. We found that incubation of isolated rat skeletal muscle with caffeine (3 mM, 15 min) has no effect on the level of tyrosine phosphorylation of IR under insulin-stimulated condition, whereas the level of tyrosine phosphorylation of IRS-1 is lower in caffeine-treated muscle compared to caffeine-untreated one. In short, it is possible that caffeine affects the functions of IRS-1 either directly and/or through molecules other than IR. In this regard, we hypothesized that the inhibitory effect of caffeine on insulin signaling and insulin-dependent glucose transport is caused by preventing IRS-1 tyrosine phosphorylation via increasing IRS-1 serine phosphorylation.

Ser^{307} of IRS-1 is located close to the phosphotyrosine-binding domain of IRS-1 [36] and its phosphorylation has been demonstrated to inhibit insulin-stimulated tyrosine phosphorylation of IRS-1 and subsequent activation of PI3K [37, 38]. We found that caffeine upregulated both basal and insulin-stimulated phosphorylation of IRS-1 Ser^{307} (Figure 2A) and phosphorylation (activation) of IκB kinase (IKK), a kinase for IRS-1 Ser^{307} [39, 40] (Figure 2B).

Moreover, the pharmacological blockade of IKK by caffeic acid alleviated the caffeine-induced insulin resistance, including IRS-1 tyrosine phosphorylation (Figure 2C), Akt phosphorylation (Figure 2D), and glucose transport (Figure 2E). Given that IKK is the master regulator of nuclear factor-kappa B (NF-κB) activation in response to inflammatory stimuli, and that the IKK/NF-κB pathway is a core mechanism that conveys insulin resistance in peripheral tissues [29, 41], it is suggested that the inhibitory effect of caffeine on insulin signaling pathways in skeletal muscle is caused by IKK-induced upregulation of IRS-1 Ser^{307} phosphorylation.

It is also suggested that Ser^{789} residue of IRS-1 plays an important role in attenuating insulin signaling and that this site is regulated by 5'AMP-activated protein kinase (AMPK) [42-44], a crucial modulator for energy homeostasis [45]. We found that caffeine increased both basal and insulin-stimulated IRS-1 Ser^{789} phosphorylation with similar increases in AMPK phosphorylation (activation).

However, our data demonstrated that suppression of AMPK phosphorylation and IRS-1 Ser^{789} phosphorylation by Ca^{2+} release blocker dantrolene, which has been reported to inhibit caffeine-induced AMPK activation in mouse skeletal muscle [46], did not rescue IRS-1 tyrosine phosphorylation, Akt phosphorylation, and insulin-stimulated glucose transport.

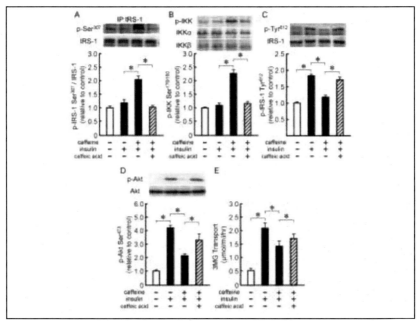

Adapted from Egawa et al. [35] with permission by the publisher.

Figure 2. The effect of caffeine on (A) IRS-1 Ser^{307} phosphorylation (p-Ser^{307}), (B) IKK Ser$^{176/180}$ phosphorylation (p-IKK), (C) IRS-1 Tyr^{612} phosphorylation (p-Tyr^{612}), (D) Akt phosphorylation (p-Akt), and (E) 3-O-methyl-D-glucose (3MG) transport. Isolated muscle was preincubated for 40 min and incubated for 15 min in the absence or presence of 3 mM caffeine. Muscle was then incubated with or without 1 μM insulin in the absence or presence of 3 mM caffeine for 15 min. When present, 5 mM caffeic acid was added throughout the preincubation and incubation periods. The tissue lysate (B-D) and immnoprecipitate by anti IRS-1 antibody (IP:IRS-1) (A) was subjected to western blot analysis. Muscle was also subjected to 3MG transport assay (E). Fold increases are expressed relative to the level of signal in the control muscles. Representative immunoblots are shown. Values are mean ± SE; n = 6-8 per group. *P<0.05.

These observations are consistent with previous data presented by Kolnes et al. [47], showing that dantrolene does not rescue caffeine-mediated blockade of insulin-stimulated Akt phosphorylation and glucose transport in incubated rat skeletal muscles. Taken together, it is suggested that caffeine inhibits insulin signaling via Ca^{2+}-independent and AMPK/IRS-1 Ser^{789}-independent mechanisms in skeletal muscle. These findings are not surprising because muscle contraction, a physiological stimulator of both Ca^{2+} release and AMPK activity, does not induce insulin resistance in skeletal muscle.

Next, to determine whether a physiological blood concentration of caffeine affects insulin signaling, the tyrosine phosphorylation of IRS-1 and phosphorylation of Akt in muscles dissected 60 min after intravenous injection of 5 mg/kg caffeine was estimated.

In humans, plasma caffeine levels reach 20–50 μM [48] following an ingestion of caffeine in amounts corresponding to 2–3 cups of coffee. Habitual coffee consumers (7 cups/day) show a peak plasma caffeine concentration of about 50 μM, with a mean 24 h plasma level of about 25 μM [49]. We previously showed that administration of 5 mg/kg caffeine into the tail vein of the rats increases the blood concentration of caffeine to 50 μM 60 min after the injection [50].

In this condition, caffeine suppressed basal and insulin-stimulated tyrosine phosphorylation of IRS-1 and phosphorylation of Akt [35]. Therefore, we speculate that caffeine-induced insulin resistance after consumption of a physiological dose of caffeine is caused by IRS-1 dysfunction, perhaps through IRS-1 Ser^{307} phosphorylation led by IKK (Figure 3).

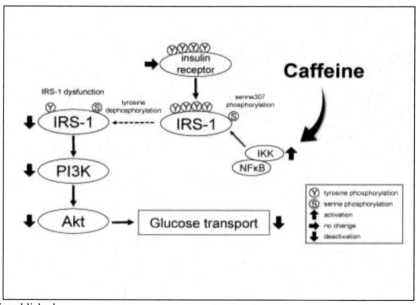

Unpublished.

Figure 3. Potential mechanism of inhibiting insulin-dependent glucose transport by caffeine in skeletal muscle.

CAFFEINE-INDUCED PROMOTION OF INSULIN-INDEPENDENT GLUCOSE TRANSPORT PATHWAY

Insulin-Independent Glucose Transport in Skeletal Muscle

In contrast to insulin, contraction does not have an influence about tyrosine phosphorylation of IR and IRS-1 and on PI3K activity [51]. In addition, muscle-specific knockout of the IR does not impair contraction-stimulated glucose transport [52]. The blockade of PI3K activity by pharmacological inhibitor wortmannin or LY294002 suppresses contraction-stimulated Akt phosphorylation and activity [53], whereas it does not inhibit contraction-stimulated GLUT4 translocation and glucose transport [54, 55]. These findings indicate that the GLUT4 translocation and glucose transport by insulin and contraction in skeletal muscles are controlled via different mechanisms.

AMPK and Insulin-Independent Glucose Transport in Skeletal Muscle

AMPK has been identified as part of the mechanisms that lead to insulin-independent glucose transport (Figure 1). AMPK is a heterotrimeric kinase comprising a catalytic α-subunit and two regulatory subunits, β and γ [56]. There are two distinct α-isoforms ($\alpha 1$ and $\alpha 2$): $\alpha 1$ is expressed ubiquitously, whereas $\alpha 2$ is dominant in skeletal muscle, heart, and liver. AMP binding to the Bateman domains of the γ-subunit of AMPK leads the allosteric activation of AMPK and phosphorylation of the Thr^{172} residue of the α-subunit, which is indispensable for maximal kinase activity. The level of phosphorylation depends on the balance of activities of upstream kinases including LKB1 and Ca^{2+}/calmodulin dependent protein kinase kinase (CaMKK) and protein phosphatases [57, 58].

AMPK classically works as a signaling intermediary in muscle cells by monitoring cellular energy status, such as the AMP/ATP ratio, and the creatine/creatine phosphate (PCr) ratio [56]. In isolated rat skeletal muscle incubated in vitro, both AMPK$\alpha 1$ and AMPK$\alpha 2$ are activated in response to energy-depriving stresses such as contraction, hypoxia, hyperosmolarity, inhibition of oxidative phosphorylation, and inhibition of electron transport [59], all of which are strong stimulators of insulin-independent glucose transport. Activation of AMPK causes the phosphorylation of multiple downstream substrates which seem to increase ATP production by activating pathways that are involved in glucose transport and fatty acid oxidation, and to simultaneously decrease ATP consumption by inhibiting pathways that lead to fatty acid, protein, and glycogen synthesis [56-58].

Caffeine and AMPK Activation in Skeletal Muscle

Early studies showed that stimulation with caffeine acutely increased insulin-independent glucose transport without apparently increasing AMPKα Thr^{172} phosphorylation in incubated rodent skeletal muscles [46, 60, 61]. On the other hand, Jensen et al. [46] showed that insulin-independent glucose transport in response to caffeine is not induced in isolated soleus muscle from AMPK kinase dead (AMPK-KD) mice.

Jensen et al. also demonstrated that caffeine acutely stimulates AMPKα1 activity, but not α2 activity, in incubated mouse and rat soleus muscles. In contrast, Raney and Turcotte [62] demonstrated that caffeine increases AMPKα2 activity in perfused rat hind limb muscles. In this way, it was not established whether caffeine activates AMPK and which the α isoform is activated if AMPK is activated.

The causation that the different observations are produced might be a muscle incubation procedure. We demonstrated previously that AMPK (mainly AMPKα1) is activated immediately as a postmortem artifact during the dissection procedure [63], so we should measure AMPK activity after a preincubation period (40 min) that was sufficient to reduce AMPK activity to the basal level. However, the preceding studies did not set a preincubation period for isolated muscles before caffeine stimulation. The actual AMPK activation may be increased by caffeine, but it may also be disturbed by additional activation during isolation because an increase in AMPK activity would be detectable only when the activation by caffeine exceeds that of the isolating stimuli.

Therefore, we thought that a preincubation period after isolation of muscle is indispensable to detect actual action of caffeine on skeletal muscle AMPK activation, and reexamined whether caffeine has the ability to stimulate AMPK in skeletal muscle setting a preincubation period [64]. We found that incubation with caffeine (≥ 3 mM, ≥ 15 min) after a preincubation period (40 min) clearly increased AMPKα Thr^{172} phosphorylation and AMPKα1 and α2 activities in rat skeletal muscles, and these were accompanied with increased indicators of AMPK activity in vivo, phosphorylation of acetyl-CoA carboxylase (ACC), an endogenous substrate of AMPK, and insulin-independent glucose transport activity.

Caffeine-induced AMPK activation was also accompanied with a reduction in fuel status of skeletal muscle. The PCr content was 23% lower in muscle stimulated with caffeine than that of the control. From these results, we judged that caffeine is capable of activating AMPK (enhancing AMPKα Thr^{172} phosphorylation) with reducing the intracellular energy status in skeletal muscle.

It is accepted that AMPK activity is regulated via both energy-dependent [65, 66] and -independent [67-69] mechanisms. We showed that caffeine-induced AMPK activation, both AMPKα1 and AMPKα2, was accompanied with energy deprivation [64].

In contrast, Jensen et al. [46] demonstrated predominant activation of AMPKα1 by caffeine but did not detect any changes in energy status. AMPKα2 has greater energy dependence than AMPKα1 in terms of the allosteric activation by AMP and covalent activation by upstream kinases [70, 71]. In support of this, we had demonstrated previously that AMPKα1, but not AMPKα2, is activated in rat epitrochlearis muscles treated with H_2O_2 and hypoxanthine/xanthine oxidase in the absence of an increase in AMP or a decrease in PCr content [72]. We had also shown that AMPKα1 is activated in low-intensity contracting muscle in which AMP concentration is not elevated, whereas AMPKα1 and α2 are activated in high-intensity contracting muscle, in which the AMP concentration is significantly higher than the resting value [63].

These findings raise the possibility that there are different pathways, energy-dependent and -independent, in caffeine-induced AMPK activation. Thus, we next investigated the effects of caffeine at lower concentrations (< 3 mM) on AMPKα1 and α2 activities in rat skeletal muscles stimulated by caffeine in vitro and in vivo [50].

We found that in vitro caffeine treatment at 1 mM activated AMPKα1 but not AMPKα2, and caffeine at 3 mM stimulated both isoforms (Figure 4A). The activation of AMPKα1 by caffeine occurred in the absence of an apparent reduction in muscle energy status (Figure 4B), and was associated with increased ACC phosphorylation and insulin-independent glucose transport activity (Figure 4C). The predominant activation of AMPKα1 was also confirmed by in vivo caffeine treatment.

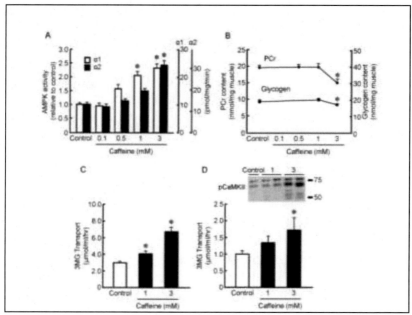

Adapted from Egawa et al. [50] with permission by the publisher.

Figure 4. The effect of caffeine on (A) AMPK activity, (B) PCr and glycogen content, (C) 3MG transport, (D) CaMKII Thr^{287} phosphorylation (pCaMKII). Isolated muscle was preincubated for 40 min and incubated for 15 min in the absence or presence of 1 or 3 mM caffeine. The tissue lysate was subjected to western blot analysis. Muscle was also subjected to 3MG transport assay. The phosphorylation of CaMKII isoforms migrated between 50 to 75 KDa was summed. Fold increases are expressed relative to the level of signal in the control muscles. Representative immunoblots are shown. Values are mean ± SE; n = 4-9 per group. *P<0.05.

Injection of 5 mg/kg of caffeine into the rat tail vein increased the blood concentration of caffeine to 50 μM (10 μg/ml) 60 min after the injection, and significantly activated AMPKα1 but not AMPKα2.

Collectively, our findings suggest that caffeine at low concentrations preferentially activates AMPKα1 in the absence of energy deprivation, and that caffeine at high concentrations activates both AMPKα1 and AMPKα2 in the presence of energy deprivation in rat skeletal muscle. It also suggests that activation of both the α1 and α2 isoforms increases insulin-independent glucose transport in skeletal muscle (Figure 5). Furthermore, we suggest that AMPKα1 plays a pivotal role in insulin-independent glucose transport in physiological conditions.

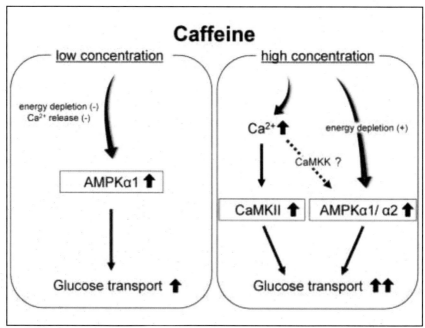

Unpublished.

Figure 5. Potential mechanism of activating insulin-independent glucose transport by caffeine in skeletal muscle.

Ca^{2+} and Insulin-Independent Glucose Transport in Skeletal Muscle

It is assumed that intracellular free Ca^{2+} in skeletal muscle plays important roles in both excitation–contraction coupling and cellular signal transduction as a second messenger that controls a variety of essential cellular functions, including insulin-independent glucose transport. Because caffeine is a major substrate that induces the release of Ca^{2+} from the sarcoplasmic reticulum, it has been used by many researchers to study the effect of Ca^{2+} signaling on skeletal muscle glucose metabolism [46, 60, 61, 73-78]. With one exception [76], it was shown that caffeine increased the insulin-independent glucose transport in skeletal muscle, and some researchers suggested that this action was led by Ca^{2+}-mediated activation of Ca^{2+}/calmodulin-dependent protein kinase (CaMK) II [60, 61] or AMPK [46, 78].

There are several CaMKs (i.e. CaMKI, CaMKII, and CaMKIV) expressed in tissues, and CaMKII is the predominant CaMK isoform that is activated by caffeine in skeletal muscle [61, 79]. Incubation of rat skeletal muscles with Ca^{2+}/calmodulin competitive inhibitors, KN-62 or KN-93 inhibits caffeine-stimulated glucose transport in the absence of insulin [61, 77] and inhibits CaMKII Thr^{287} phosphorylation [61], an indicator of CaMKII activation. We also found that high concentrations of caffeine (3 mM) promoted CaMKII Thr^{287} phosphorylation, but low concentrations of caffeine (1 mM) did not (Figure 4D), although both of them increased insulin-independent glucose transport (Figure 4C). CaMKII and AMPK are considered to be involved in distinct signaling pathways regulated by Ca^{2+}/calmodulin, and thus both CaMKII and AMPK pathways are suggested to be involved in promoting insulin-independent glucose transport in response to stimulation with caffeine (especially high concentration) (Figure 5).

As described above, AMPK is activated by the phosphorylation of a specific site at Thr^{172} via upstream kinases, such as CaMKK. CaMKK is a major kinase, which is activated by an increase in intracellular Ca^{2+} concentration [80], and does not interact with CaMKII. It was reported that caffeine-induced AMPK activation was blocked by a CaMKK inhibitor in rodent skeletal muscle [46] and that caffeine enhanced the phosphorylation of CaMKI, which is a downstream target of CaMKK [78]. On the other hand, we found that caffeine-induced AMPKα Thr^{172} phosphorylation was abolished by incubation with Ca^{2+} releaser, dantrolene [35], but CaMKI phosphorylation did not occur by caffeine stimulation in rat skeletal muscle [50]. Taken together, we suggest that caffeine-induced Ca^{2+} release stimulates both AMPK and CaMKII, thereby stimulating insulin-independent glucose transport, and activation of AMPK by caffeine is partly via some Ca^{2+}-dependent pathway other than CaMKII (Figure 5). Further study is needed to clear the association between AMPK and CaMKK during caffeine stimulation.

CONCLUSION AND PERSPECTIVES

Caffeine is one of most widely consumed phytochemicals in the world. Therefore, to resolve the paradoxical effect of caffeine on glucose metabolism can be conducive to health promotion, especially prevention of T2DM. In the present chapter, we introduced the molecular mechanisms of caffeine for acutely regulating insulin-dependent and insulin-independent glucose transport in skeletal muscle. First, we confirmed that caffeine inhibited insulin-dependent glucose transport, and found that this was attributed to IRS-1 dysfunction led by IKK-induced phosphorylation of IRS-1 Ser^{307}. We insist that this functional loss of IRS-1 is one of causation; that ingestion of caffeine acutely impairs skeletal muscle insulin sensitivity or even whole-body glucose tolerance. On the other hand, several reports have been shown that caffeine acutely enhances insulin-independent glucose transport and activates AMPK in skeletal muscle, and we found that this activation effect was similar to that occurred by muscle contraction in terms of energy-independent and predominant activation of AMPKα1. Skeletal muscle AMPK is implicated in a variety of antidiabetic properties of exercise, including enhanced insulin-independent glucose transport [54, 59, 81], insulin sensitivity [82-87], GLUT4 expression [86, 88, 89], fatty acid oxidation [90-92] via the inhibition of ACC, modulation of glycogen synthesis [93-95] and mitochondrial biogenesis via peroxisome proliferator-activated receptor-γ coactivator 1α (PGC1α) [96, 97] and SIRT1 [98], and alterations in the distribution of muscle fiber types [99]. In addition, our study [50] and previous studies [60, 61] have shown that caffeine has the ability to activate CaMKII. It was recently reported that CaMKII plays an important role in regulating GLUT4 expression [100], and thus activation of CaMKII possibly contributes to enhancement of skeletal muscle insulin sensitivity.

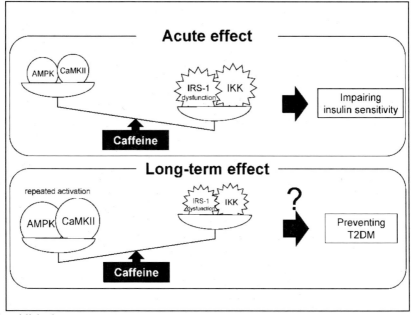

Unpublished.

Figure 6. Proposed mechanism of preventing T2DM by caffeine.

Collectively, caffeine has the potential to enhance skeletal muscle and whole-body glucose metabolism via activation of AMPK and CaMKII. We speculate that, through repeated activation of AMPK and CaMKII, long-term consumption of caffeine overcomes the simultaneous negative effect in impairing insulin sensitivity, thereby ultimately preventing T2DM (Figure 6). Further research, especially into chronic caffeine use, is required to clarify whether caffeine is a beneficial phytochemical in reducing the risk of T2DM.

REFERENCES

[1] Wild S., Roglic G., Green A., Sicree R., and King H. (2004). Global prevalence of diabetes: estimates for the year 2000 and projections for 2030. *Diabetes Care*, 27, 1047-1053.

[2] Shaw J. E., Sicree R. A., and Zimmet P. Z. (2010). Global estimates of the prevalence of diabetes for 2010 and 2030. *Diabetes Res. Clin. Pract.*, 87, 4-14.

[3] Yang W., Lu J., Weng J., Jia W., Ji L., Xiao J., Shan Z., Liu J., Tian H., Ji Q., Zhu D., Ge J., Lin L., Chen L., Guo X., Zhao Z., Li Q., Zhou Z., Shan G., He J., China National D., and Metabolic Disorders Study G. (2010). Prevalence of diabetes among men and women in China. *N. Engl. J. Med.*, 362, 1090-1101.

[4] Zhang P., Zhang X., Brown J., Vistisen D., Sicree R., Shaw J., and Nichols G. (2010). Global healthcare expenditure on diabetes for 2010 and 2030. *Diabetes Res. Clin. Pract.*, 87, 293-301.

[5] Jiang X., Zhang D., and Jiang W. (2014). Coffee and caffeine intake and incidence of type 2 diabetes mellitus: a meta-analysis of prospective studies. *Eur. J. Nutr.*, 53, 25-38.

[6] Iso H., Date C., Wakai K., Fukui M., Tamakoshi A., and Group J. S. (2006). The relationship between green tea and total caffeine intake and risk for self-reported type 2 diabetes among Japanese adults. *Ann. Intern. Med.*, 144, 554-562.

[7] Park S., Jang J. S., and Hong S. M. (2007). Long-term consumption of caffeine improves glucose homeostasis by enhancing insulinotropic action through islet insulin/insulin-like growth factor 1 signaling in diabetic rats. *Metabolism*, 56, 599-607.

[8] Lopez-Garcia E., van Dam R. M., Rajpathak S., Willett W. C., Manson J. E., and Hu F. B. (2006). Changes in caffeine intake and long-term weight change in men and women. *Am. J. Clin. Nutr.*, 83, 674-680.

[9] Williams C. J., Fargnoli J. L., Hwang J. J., van Dam R. M., Blackburn G. L., Hu F. B., and Mantzoros C. S. (2008). Coffee consumption is associated with higher plasma adiponectin concentrations in women with or without type 2 diabetes: a prospective cohort study. *Diabetes Care*, 31, 504-507.

[10] Yamauchi R., Kobayashi M., Matsuda Y., Ojika M., Shigeoka S., Yamamoto Y., Tou Y., Inoue T., Katagiri T., Murai A., and Horio F. (2010). Coffee and caffeine ameliorate hyperglycemia, fatty liver, and inflammatory adipocytokine expression in spontaneously diabetic KK-Ay mice. *J. Agric. Food Chem.*, 58, 5597-5603.

[11] Matsuda Y., Kobayashi M., Yamauchi R., Ojika M., Hiramitsu M., Inoue T., Katagiri T., Murai A., and Horio F. (2011). Coffee and caffeine improve insulin sensitivity and glucose tolerance in C57BL/6J mice fed a high-fat diet. *Biosci. Biotechnol. Biochem.*, 75, 2309-2315.

[12] Yeh T. C., Liu C. P., Cheng W. H., Chen B. R., Lu P. J., Cheng P. W., Ho W. Y., Sun G. C., Liou J. C., and Tseng C. J. (2014). Caffeine Intake Improves Fructose-Induced Hypertension and Insulin Resistance by Enhancing Central Insulin Signaling. *Hypertension*, 63, 535-541.

[13] Battram D. S., Graham T. E., Richter E. A., and Dela F. (2005). The effect of caffeine on glucose kinetics in humans--influence of adrenaline. *J. Physiol.*, 569, 347-355.

[14] Greer F., Hudson R., Ross R., and Graham T. (2001). Caffeine ingestion decreases glucose disposal during a hyperinsulinemic-euglycemic clamp in sedentary humans. *Diabetes*, 50, 2349-2354.

[15] Lane J. D., Barkauskas C. E., Surwit R. S., and Feinglos M. N. (2004). Caffeine impairs glucose metabolism in type 2 diabetes. *Diabetes Care*, 27, 2047-2048.

[16] Lee S., Hudson R., Kilpatrick K., Graham T. E., and Ross R. (2005). Caffeine ingestion is associated with reductions in glucose uptake independent of obesity and type 2 diabetes before and after exercise training. *Diabetes Care*, 28, 566-572.

[17] Petrie H. J., Chown S. E., Belfie L. M., Duncan A. M., McLaren D. H., Conquer J. A., and Graham T. E. (2004). Caffeine ingestion increases the insulin response to an oral-glucose-tolerance test in obese men before and after weight loss. *Am. J. Clin. Nutr.*, 80, 22-28.

[18] Robinson L. E., Savani S., Battram D. S., McLaren D. H., Sathasivam P., and Graham T. E. (2004). Caffeine ingestion before an oral glucose tolerance test impairs blood glucose management in men with type 2 diabetes. *J. Nutr.*, 134, 2528-2533.

[19] Beaudoin M. S., Allen B., Mazzetti G., Sullivan P. J., and Graham T. E. (2013). Caffeine ingestion impairs insulin sensitivity in a dose-dependent manner in both men and women. *Appl. Physiol. Nutr. Metab.*, 38, 140-147.

[20] Cline G. W., Petersen K. F., Krssak M., Shen J., Hundal R. S., Trajanoski Z., Inzucchi S., Dresner A., Rothman D. L., and Shulman G. I. (1999). Impaired glucose transport as a cause of decreased insulin-stimulated muscle glycogen synthesis in type 2 diabetes. *N. Engl. J. Med.*, 341, 240-246.

[21] DeFronzo R. A., Gunnarsson R., Bjorkman O., Olsson M., and Wahren J. (1985). Effects of insulin on peripheral and splanchnic glucose metabolism in noninsulin-dependent (type II) diabetes mellitus. *J. Clin. Invest.*, 76, 149-155.

[22] Kennedy J. W., Hirshman M. F., Gervino E. V., Ocel J. V., Forse R. A., Hoenig S. J., Aronson D., Goodyear L. J., and Horton E. S. (1999). Acute exercise induces GLUT4 translocation in skeletal muscle of normal human subjects and subjects with type 2 diabetes. *Diabetes*, 48, 1192-1197.

[23] Hayashi T., Wojtaszewski J. F., and Goodyear L. J. (1997). Exercise regulation of glucose transport in skeletal muscle. *Am. J. Physiol.*, 273, E1039-1051.

[24] Treebak J. T., Pehmoller C., Kristensen J. M., Kjobsted R., Birk J. B., Schjerling P., Richter E. A., Goodyear L. J., and Wojtaszewski J. F. (2014). Acute exercise and physiological insulin induce distinct phosphorylation signatures on TBC1D1 and TBC1D4 in human skeletal muscle. *J. Physiol.*, 592, 351-375.

[25] Sesti G., Federici M., Hribal M. L., Lauro D., Sbraccia P., and Lauro R. (2001). Defects of the insulin receptor substrate (IRS) system in human metabolic disorders. *Faseb. J.*, 15, 2099-2111.

[26] Smith U. (2002). Impaired ('diabetic') insulin signaling and action occur in fat cells long before glucose intolerance--is insulin resistance initiated in the adipose tissue? *Int. J. Obes. Relat. Metab. Disord.*, 26, 897-904.

[27] Gual P., Le Marchand-Brustel Y., and Tanti J. F. (2005). Positive and negative regulation of insulin signaling through IRS-1 phosphorylation. *Biochimie*, 87, 99-109.

[28] Boura-Halfon S. and Zick Y. (2009). Phosphorylation of IRS proteins, insulin action, and insulin resistance. *Am. J. Physiol. Endocrinol. Metab.*, 296, E581-591.

[29] Tanti J. F. and Jager J. (2009). Cellular mechanisms of insulin resistance: role of stress-regulated serine kinases and insulin receptor substrates (IRS) serine phosphorylation. *Curr. Opin. Pharmacol.*, 9, 753-762.

[30] Abdul-Ghani M. A. and DeFronzo R. A. (2010). Pathogenesis of insulin resistance in skeletal muscle. *J. Biomed. Biotechnol.*, 2010, 476279.

[31] Yu C., Chen Y., Cline G. W., Zhang D., Zong H., Wang Y., Bergeron R., Kim J. K., Cushman S. W., Cooney G. J., Atcheson B., White M. F., Kraegen E. W., and Shulman G. I. (2002). Mechanism by which fatty acids inhibit insulin activation of insulin receptor substrate-1 (IRS-1)-associated phosphatidylinositol 3-kinase activity in muscle. *J. Biol. Chem.*, 277, 50230-50236.

[32] Morino K., Petersen K. F., Dufour S., Befroy D., Frattini J., Shatzkes N., Neschen S., White M. F., Bilz S., Sono S., Pypaert M., and Shulman G. I. (2005). Reduced mitochondrial density and increased IRS-1 serine phosphorylation in muscle of insulin-resistant offspring of type 2 diabetic parents. *J. Clin. Invest.*, 115, 3587-3593.

[33] Keijzers G. B., De Galan B. E., Tack C. J., and Smits P. (2002). Caffeine can decrease insulin sensitivity in humans. *Diabetes Care*, 25, 364-369.

[34] Thong F. S., Derave W., Kiens B., Graham T. E., Urso B., Wojtaszewski J. F., Hansen B. F., and Richter E. A. (2002). Caffeine-induced impairment of insulin action but not insulin signaling in human skeletal muscle is reduced by exercise. *Diabetes,* 51, 583-590.

[35] Egawa T., Tsuda S., Ma X., Hamada T., and Hayashi T. (2011). Caffeine modulates phosphorylation of insulin receptor substrate-1 and impairs insulin signal transduction in rat skeletal muscle. *J. Appl. Physiol.*, 111, 1629-1636.

[36] Taniguchi C. M., Emanuelli B., and Kahn C. R. (2006). Critical nodes in signalling pathways: insights into insulin action. *Nat. Rev. Mol. Cell Biol.*, 7, 85-96.

[37] Aguirre V., Werner E. D., Giraud J., Lee Y. H., Shoelson S. E., and White M. F. (2002). Phosphorylation of Ser307 in insulin receptor substrate-1 blocks interactions with the insulin receptor and inhibits insulin action. *J. Biol. Chem.*, 277, 1531-1537.

[38] Hirosumi J., Tuncman G., Chang L., Gorgun C. Z., Uysal K. T., Maeda K., Karin M., and Hotamisligil G. S. (2002). A central role for JNK in obesity and insulin resistance. *Nature,* 420, 333-336.

[39] de Alvaro C., Teruel T., Hernandez R., and Lorenzo M. (2004). Tumor necrosis factor alpha produces insulin resistance in skeletal muscle by

activation of inhibitor kappaB kinase in a p38 MAPK-dependent manner. *J. Biol. Chem.*, 279, 17070-17078.

[40] Gao Z., Hwang D., Bataille F., Lefevre M., York D., Quon M. J., and Ye J. (2002). Serine phosphorylation of insulin receptor substrate 1 by inhibitor kappa B kinase complex. *J. Biol. Chem.*, 277, 48115-48121.

[41] Shoelson S. E., Lee J., and Yuan M. (2003). Inflammation and the IKK beta/I kappa B/NF-kappa B axis in obesity- and diet-induced insulin resistance. *Int. J. Obes. Relat. Metab. Disord.*, 27 Suppl 3, S49-52.

[42] Qiao L. Y., Zhande R., Jetton T. L., Zhou G., and Sun X. J. (2002). In vivo phosphorylation of insulin receptor substrate 1 at serine 789 by a novel serine kinase in insulin-resistant rodents. *J. Biol. Chem.*, 277, 26530-26539.

[43] Horike N., Takemori H., Katoh Y., Doi J., Min L., Asano T., Sun X. J., Yamamoto H., Kasayama S., Muraoka M., Nonaka Y., and Okamoto M. (2003). Adipose-specific expression, phosphorylation of Ser794 in insulin receptor substrate-1, and activation in diabetic animals of salt-inducible kinase-2. *J. Biol. Chem.*, 278, 18440-18447.

[44] Tzatsos A. and Tsichlis P. N. (2007). Energy depletion inhibits phosphatidylinositol 3-kinase/Akt signaling and induces apoptosis via AMP-activated protein kinase-dependent phosphorylation of IRS-1 at Ser-794. *J. Biol. Chem.*, 282, 18069-18082.

[45] Hardie D. G. (2011). Energy sensing by the AMP-activated protein kinase and its effects on muscle metabolism. *Proc. Nutr. Soc.*, 70, 92-99.

[46] Jensen T. E., Rose A. J., Hellsten Y., Wojtaszewski J. F., and Richter E. A. (2007). Caffeine-induced Ca(2+) release increases AMPK-dependent glucose uptake in rodent soleus muscle. *Am. J. Physiol. Endocrinol. Metab.*, 293, E286-292.

[47] Kolnes A. J., Ingvaldsen A., Bolling A., Stuenaes J. T., Kreft M., Zorec R., Shepherd P. R., and Jensen J. (2010). Caffeine and theophylline block insulin-stimulated glucose uptake and PKB phosphorylation in rat skeletal muscles. *Acta. Physiol. (Oxf)*, 200, 65-74.

[48] Fredholm B. B. (1980). Are methylxanthine effects due to antagonism of endogenous adenosine? *Trends in Pharmacological Sciences*, 1, 129-132.

[49] Lelo A., Miners J. O., Robson R., and Birkett D. J. (1986). Assessment of caffeine exposure: caffeine content of beverages, caffeine intake, and plasma concentrations of methylxanthines. *Clin. Pharmacol. Ther.*, 39, 54-59.

[50] Egawa T., Hamada T., Ma X., Karaike K., Kameda N., Masuda S., Iwanaka N., and Hayashi T. (2011). Caffeine activates preferentially alpha1-isoform of 5'AMP-activated protein kinase in rat skeletal muscle. *Acta. Physiol. (Oxf)*, 201, 227-238.

[51] Goodyear L. J., Giorgino F., Balon T. W., Condorelli G., and Smith R. J. (1995). Effects of contractile activity on tyrosine phosphoproteins and PI 3-kinase activity in rat skeletal muscle. *Am. J. Physiol.*, 268, E987-995.

[52] Wojtaszewski J. F., Higaki Y., Hirshman M. F., Michael M. D., Dufresne S. D., Kahn C. R., and Goodyear L. J. (1999). Exercise modulates postreceptor insulin signaling and glucose transport in muscle-specific insulin receptor knockout mice. *J. Clin. Invest.*, 104, 1257-1264.

[53] Sakamoto K., Hirshman M. F., Aschenbach W. G., and Goodyear L. J. (2002). Contraction regulation of Akt in rat skeletal muscle. *J. Biol. Chem.*, 277, 11910-11917.

[54] Hayashi T., Hirshman M. F., Kurth E. J., Winder W. W., and Goodyear L. J. (1998). Evidence for 5' AMP-activated protein kinase mediation of the effect of muscle contraction on glucose transport. *Diabetes*, 47, 1369-1373.

[55] Lund S., Holman G. D., Schmitz O., and Pedersen O. (1995). Contraction stimulates translocation of glucose transporter GLUT4 in skeletal muscle through a mechanism distinct from that of insulin. *Proc. Natl. Acad. Sci. U S A*, 92, 5817-5821.

[56] Hardie D. G. and Carling D. (1997). The AMP-activated protein kinase--fuel gauge of the mammalian cell? *Eur. J. Biochem.*, 246, 259-273.

[57] Fogarty S. and Hardie D. G. (2010). Development of protein kinase activators: AMPK as a target in metabolic disorders and cancer. *Biochim. Biophys. Acta.*, 1804, 581-591.

[58] Witczak C. A., Sharoff C. G., and Goodyear L. J. (2008). AMP-activated protein kinase in skeletal muscle: from structure and localization to its role as a master regulator of cellular metabolism. *Cell Mol. Life Sci.*, 65, 3737-3755.

[59] Hayashi T., Hirshman M. F., Fujii N., Habinowski S. A., Witters L. A., and Goodyear L. J. (2000). Metabolic stress and altered glucose transport: activation of AMP-activated protein kinase as a unifying coupling mechanism. *Diabetes*, 49, 527-531.

[60] Canto C., Chibalin A. V., Barnes B. R., Glund S., Suarez E., Ryder J. W., Palacin M., Zierath J. R., Zorzano A., and Guma A. (2006).

Neuregulins mediate calcium-induced glucose transport during muscle contraction. *J. Biol. Chem.*, 281, 21690-21697.

[61] Wright D. C., Hucker K. A., Holloszy J. O., and Han D. H. (2004). Ca2+ and AMPK both mediate stimulation of glucose transport by muscle contractions. *Diabetes,* 53, 330-335.

[62] Raney M. A. and Turcotte L. P. (2008). Evidence for the involvement of CaMKII and AMPK in Ca2+-dependent signaling pathways regulating FA uptake and oxidation in contracting rodent muscle. *J. Appl. Physiol.*, 104, 1366-1373.

[63] Toyoda T., Tanaka S., Ebihara K., Masuzaki H., Hosoda K., Sato K., Fushiki T., Nakao K., and Hayashi T. (2006). Low-intensity contraction activates the alpha1-isoform of 5'-AMP-activated protein kinase in rat skeletal muscle. *Am. J. Physiol. Endocrinol. Metab.*, 290, E583-590.

[64] Egawa T., Hamada T., Kameda N., Karaike K., Ma X., Masuda S., Iwanaka N., and Hayashi T. (2009). Caffeine acutely activates 5'adenosine monophosphate-activated protein kinase and increases insulin-independent glucose transport in rat skeletal muscles. *Metabolism,* 58, 1609-1617.

[65] Hawley S. A., Boudeau J., Reid J. L., Mustard K. J., Udd L., Makela T. P., Alessi D. R., and Hardie D. G. (2003). Complexes between the LKB1 tumor suppressor, STRAD alpha/beta and MO25 alpha/beta are upstream kinases in the AMP-activated protein kinase cascade. *J. Biol.*, 2, 28.

[66] Sakamoto K., Goransson O., Hardie D. G., and Alessi D. R. (2004). Activity of LKB1 and AMPK-related kinases in skeletal muscle: effects of contraction, phenformin, and AICAR. *Am. J. Physiol. Endocrinol. Metab.*, 287, E310-317.

[67] Hawley S. A., Pan D. A., Mustard K. J., Ross L., Bain J., Edelman A. M., Frenguelli B. G., and Hardie D. G. (2005). Calmodulin-dependent protein kinase kinase-beta is an alternative upstream kinase for AMP-activated protein kinase. *Cell Metab.*, 2, 9-19.

[68] Hurley R. L., Anderson K. A., Franzone J. M., Kemp B. E., Means A. R., and Witters L. A. (2005). The Ca2+/calmodulin-dependent protein kinase kinases are AMP-activated protein kinase kinases. *J. Biol. Chem.*, 280, 29060-29066.

[69] Woods A., Dickerson K., Heath R., Hong S. P., Momcilovic M., Johnstone S. R., Carlson M., and Carling D. (2005). Ca2+/calmodulin-dependent protein kinase kinase-beta acts upstream of AMP-activated protein kinase in mammalian cells. *Cell Metab.*, 2, 21-33.

[70] Salt I., Celler J. W., Hawley S. A., Prescott A., Woods A., Carling D., and Hardie D. G. (1998). AMP-activated protein kinase: greater AMP dependence, and preferential nuclear localization, of complexes containing the alpha2 isoform. *Biochem. J.*, 334, 177-187.

[71] Stein S. C., Woods A., Jones N. A., Davison M. D., and Carling D. (2000). The regulation of AMP-activated protein kinase by phosphorylation. *Biochem. J.*, 345, 437-443.

[72] Toyoda T., Hayashi T., Miyamoto L., Yonemitsu S., Nakano M., Tanaka S., Ebihara K., Masuzaki H., Hosoda K., Inoue G., Otaka A., Sato K., Fushiki T., and Nakao K. (2004). Possible involvement of the alpha1 isoform of 5'AMP-activated protein kinase in oxidative stress-stimulated glucose transport in skeletal muscle. *Am. J. Physiol. Endocrinol. Metab.*, 287, E166-173.

[73] Holloszy J. O. and Narahara H. T. (1967). Enhanced permeability to sugar associated with muscle contraction. Studies of the role of Ca++. *J. Gen. Physiol.*, 50, 551-562.

[74] Youn J. H., Gulve E. A., and Holloszy J. O. (1991). Calcium stimulates glucose transport in skeletal muscle by a pathway independent of contraction. *Am. J. Physiol.*, 260, C555-561.

[75] Cartee G. D., Douen A. G., Ramlal T., Klip A., and Holloszy J. O. (1991). Stimulation of glucose transport in skeletal muscle by hypoxia. *J. Appl. Physiol.*, 70, 1593-1600.

[76] Maclean P. S. and Winder W. W. (1995). Caffeine decreases malonyl-CoA in isolated perfused skeletal muscle of rats. *J. Appl. Physiol.*, 78, 1496-1501.

[77] Wright D. C., Geiger P. C., Holloszy J. O., and Han D. H. (2005). Contraction- and hypoxia-stimulated glucose transport is mediated by a Ca2+-dependent mechanism in slow-twitch rat soleus muscle. *Am. J. Physiol. Endocrinol. Metab.*, 288, E1062-1066.

[78] Abbott M. J., Edelman A. M., and Turcotte L. P. (2009). CaMKK is an upstream signal of AMP-activated protein kinase in regulation of substrate metabolism in contracting skeletal muscle. *Am. J. Physiol. Regul. Integr. Comp. Physiol.*, 297, R1724-1732.

[79] Rose A. J., Kiens B., and Richter E. A. (2006). Ca2+-calmodulin-dependent protein kinase expression and signalling in skeletal muscle during exercise. *J. Physiol.*, 574, 889-903.

[80] Hook S. S. and Means A. R. (2001). Ca(2+)/CaM-dependent kinases: from activation to function. *Annual review of pharmacology and toxicology*, 41, 471-505.

[81] Mu J., Brozinick J. T., Jr., Valladares O., Bucan M., and Birnbaum M. J. (2001). A role for AMP-activated protein kinase in contraction- and hypoxia-regulated glucose transport in skeletal muscle. *Mol. Cell*, 7, 1085-1094.

[82] Fiedler M., Zierath J. R., Selen G., Wallberg-Henriksson H., Liang Y., and Sakariassen K. S. (2001). 5-aminoimidazole-4-carboxy-amide-1-beta-D-ribofuranoside treatment ameliorates hyperglycaemia and hyperinsulinaemia but not dyslipidaemia in KKAy-CETP mice. *Diabetologia*, 44, 2180-2186.

[83] Iglesias M. A., Ye J. M., Frangioudakis G., Saha A. K., Tomas E., Ruderman N. B., Cooney G. J., and Kraegen E. W. (2002). AICAR administration causes an apparent enhancement of muscle and liver insulin action in insulin-resistant high-fat-fed rats. *Diabetes*, 51, 2886-2894.

[84] Buhl E. S., Jessen N., Pold R., Ledet T., Flyvbjerg A., Pedersen S. B., Pedersen O., Schmitz O., and Lund S. (2002). Long-term AICAR administration reduces metabolic disturbances and lowers blood pressure in rats displaying features of the insulin resistance syndrome. *Diabetes*, 51, 2199-2206.

[85] Pold R., Jensen L. S., Jessen N., Buhl E. S., Schmitz O., Flyvbjerg A., Fujii N., Goodyear L. J., Gotfredsen C. F., Brand C. L., and Lund S. (2005). Long-term AICAR administration and exercise prevents diabetes in ZDF rats. *Diabetes*, 54, 928-934.

[86] Nakano M., Hamada T., Hayashi T., Yonemitsu S., Miyamoto L., Toyoda T., Tanaka S., Masuzaki H., Ebihara K., Ogawa Y., Hosoda K., Inoue G., Yoshimasa Y., Otaka A., Fushiki T., and Nakao K. (2006). alpha2 isoform-specific activation of 5'adenosine monophosphate-activated protein kinase by 5-aminoimidazole-4-carboxamide-1-beta-D-ribonucleoside at a physiological level activates glucose transport and increases glucose transporter 4 in mouse skeletal muscle. *Metabolism*, 55, 300-308.

[87] Tanaka S., Hayashi T., Toyoda T., Hamada T., Shimizu Y., Hirata M., Ebihara K., Masuzaki H., Hosoda K., Fushiki T., and Nakao K. (2007). High-fat diet impairs the effects of a single bout of endurance exercise on glucose transport and insulin sensitivity in rat skeletal muscle. *Metabolism*, 56, 1719-1728.

[88] Zheng D, MacLean P. S., Pohnert S. C., Knight J. B., Olson A. L., Winder W. W., and Dohm G. L. (2001). Regulation of muscle GLUT-4

transcription by AMP-activated protein kinase. *J. Appl. Physiol.*, 91, 1073-1083.

[89] Holmes B. and Dohm G. L. (2004). Regulation of GLUT4 gene expression during exercise. *Med. Sci. Sports Exerc.*, 36, 1202-1206.

[90] Winder W. W. and Hardie D. G. (1996). Inactivation of acetyl-CoA carboxylase and activation of AMP-activated protein kinase in muscle during exercise. *Am. J. Physiol.*, 270, E299-304.

[91] Vavvas D., Apazidis A., Saha A. K., Gamble J., Patel A., Kemp B. E., Witters L. A., and Ruderman N. B. (1997). Contraction-induced changes in acetyl-CoA carboxylase and 5'-AMP-activated kinase in skeletal muscle. *J. Biol. Chem.*, 272, 13255-13261.

[92] Hutber C. A., Hardie D. G., and Winder W. W. (1997). Electrical stimulation inactivates muscle acetyl-CoA carboxylase and increases AMP-activated protein kinase. *Am. J. Physiol.*, 272, E262-266.

[93] Wojtaszewski J. F., Jorgensen S. B., Hellsten Y., Hardie D. G., and Richter E. A. (2002). Glycogen-dependent effects of 5-aminoimidazole-4-carboxamide (AICA)-riboside on AMP-activated protein kinase and glycogen synthase activities in rat skeletal muscle. *Diabetes,* 51, 284-292.

[94] Jorgensen S. B., Nielsen J. N., Birk J. B., Olsen G. S., Viollet B., Andreelli F., Schjerling P., Vaulont S., Hardie D. G., Hansen B. F., Richter E. A., and Wojtaszewski J. F. (2004). The alpha2-5'AMP-activated protein kinase is a site 2 glycogen synthase kinase in skeletal muscle and is responsive to glucose loading. *Diabetes*, 53, 3074-3081.

[95] Miyamoto L., Toyoda T., Hayashi T., Yonemitsu S., Nakano M., Tanaka S., Ebihara K., Masuzaki H., Hosoda K., Ogawa Y., Inoue G., Fushiki T., and Nakao K. (2007). Effect of acute activation of 5'-AMP-activated protein kinase on glycogen regulation in isolated rat skeletal muscle. *J. Appl. Physiol.,* 102, 1007-1013.

[96] Jager S., Handschin C., St-Pierre J., and Spiegelman B. M. (2007). AMP-activated protein kinase (AMPK) action in skeletal muscle via direct phosphorylation of PGC-1alpha. *Proc. Natl. Acad. Sci. U S A,* 104, 12017-12022.

[97] Garcia-Roves P. M., Osler M. E., Holmstrom M. H., and Zierath J. R. (2008). Gain-of-function R225Q mutation in AMP-activated protein kinase gamma3 subunit increases mitochondrial biogenesis in glycolytic skeletal muscle. *J. Biol. Chem.*, 283, 35724-35734.

[98] Canto C., Gerhart-Hines Z., Feige J. N., Lagouge M., Noriega L., Milne J. C., Elliott P. J., Puigserver P., and Auwerx J. (2009). AMPK regulates

energy expenditure by modulating NAD+ metabolism and SIRT1 activity. *Nature,* 458, 1056-1060.

[99] Rockl K. S., Hirshman M. F., Brandauer J., Fujii N., Witters L. A., and Goodyear L. J. (2007). Skeletal muscle adaptation to exercise training: AMP-activated protein kinase mediates muscle fiber type shift. *Diabetes,* 56, 2062-2069.

[100] Ojuka E. O., Goyaram V., and Smith J. A. (2012). The role of CaMKII in regulating GLUT4 expression in skeletal muscle. *Am. J. Physiol. Endocrinol. Metab.,* 303, E322-331.

[101] Egawa T., Ma X., Hamada T., and Hayashi T. (2013). Chapter 90 - Caffeine and Insulin-Independent Glucose Transport. In: Preedy VR. Tea in Health and Disease Prevention. Academic Press; 1077-1088.

In: Caffeine
Editor: Aimée S. Tolley

ISBN: 978-1-63117-777-4
© 2014 Nova Science Publishers, Inc.

Chapter 6

UTILIZATION EFFICIENCY IMPROVEMENT OF TEA LEAVES' BIOLOGICAL POTENTIAL AS A RESULT OF SC-CO$_2$ PRETREATMENT

F. M. Gumerov[1], Truong Nam Hung[2], F. N. Shamsetdinov[1], Z. I. Zaripov[1], F. R. Gabitov[1] and B. Le Neindre[3]

[1]Kazan National Research Technological University, Kazan, Russia
[2]Power University of Hanoi, Hanoi, Viet Nam
[3]LSPM CNRS, University Paris, Villetaneuse, France

ABSTRACT

The pretreatment of commercial samples of Vietnamese and Chinese green teas shows that it is possible to increase the extractability of chemical, including caffeine, in aqueous phase at the stage of beverage concoction and provide more complete information of biological potential of the feedstock. Procedures are proposed for an extract of raw materials in (SC-CO$_2$) medium; (SC-CO$_2$) circulation through the processed raw materials, multiple decompressions in (SC-CO$_2$) medium, containing processed raw materials. For example, the circulation of carbon dioxide during 4 hours through the extractor with the feedstock at $T = 333.15\,K$ and $P = 10$ MPa provides 25% increased caffeine yield, into the aqueous phase, at the stage of beverage concoction. The conditions to minimize the effect of (SC-CO$_2$) extraction, upon minerals and biologically active components of tea leaves are investigated in the implementation of these procedures In particular, the study of solubility of caffeine in supercritical carbon dioxide in the temperature range T = 308.15-333.15 K and the pressure range P = 7-30 MPa, shows that the pressure range of 7-11 MPa gives optimal results for (SC-CO_2) flowing through the processing raw materials. The results of research of the other factors, related to the procedure, and properties of the corresponding thermodynamic systems are presented; there are required for the mathematical modeling of the operating process, in order to serve as a basis for designing the future large scale equipment. In particular, the behavior of the following properties has been investigated: the enthalpy of mixing for (caffeine - SC-CO_2) systems and (cellulose - SC-CO_2) systems at 308.15K, 323.15K, 348.15K isotherms in the pressure range 0-40 MPa and 8-22 MPa, respectively. The isobaric heat capacity and density of (caffeine - carbon dioxide) mixtures; as well as some properties of the ternary system, containing (caffeine, carbon dioxide and water) are carried out. The results of the influence of the pretreatment on the composition and structure of tea leaves, cellulose and caffeine are presented. The results of solubility data and some useful properties of thermodynamic systems are reported.

1. INTRODUCTION

Russia is one of the largest manufacturing country and consumer of tea in the world. Its imports vary from 150 to 170 thousand tons of black tea and green pekoe each year. Twenty percent of this production is used as raw material for industrial processing [1]. Green tea, made from young leaves and buds unfermented, is one of the most common beverages in the world. In Western world, green tea is best known for its stimulating and refreshing as a drink, although its use in cosmetics is increasing, while in Asia, its medicinal properties have been known since antiquity. Epidemiological observations have shown a significant impact on reducing cancer and cardiovascular disease in populations with high consumption of green tea. The main active ingredients of green tea are polyphenols, methylxanthines, theanine. xanthine dominant is similar to caffeine also called theine, a stimulant and analeptic which is dose dependent. All green teas such as Camellia sinesis, contain more or less the same amount of caffeine, usually 3–6 wt. %.Even if the caffeine content in green tea leaf is larger than in coffee bean, one cup of green tea contains less caffeine than a cup of coffee, because tea is brewed normally at much lower temperature. Furthermore, tannin in green tea alters the action of caffeine in the body, because caffeine is absorbed more slowly in the body during a longer period of time.

Today, most approaches and methods of processing green tea leaves are related to decaffeination. They are similar to those used for the decaffeination of coffee. Several methods of decaffeination of tea are known. They deal in part, with the manufacture of decaffeinated tea leaves, and in part, with the manufacture of instant tea powder without caffeine [2]. The decaffeination of tea is usually done on a dried fermented product which makes it extremely sensitive to a change in its flavor. For example, an aqueous extract of decaffeinated tea was produced by the method of brewing with a solvent for caffeine immiscible with water, whereupon the first tea ex-tract has been impregnated with the concentrated extract caffeine-free and dried. In another method, the aromatic substances are first removed from the tea using petroleum ether. The tea is then moistened, and then the caffeine is extracted with other solvents. After drying the tea, aromatic substances that were originally removed from the tea is added to tea again. In a method similar aromatic substances are extracted with a solvent having a low boiling point, such as trichloroethylene, the extraction of caffeine is produced by a solvent with high boiling point, as tetra-chloride carbon, after treatment with alcoholic ammonia solution. All these methods have several disadvantages, because they use, among others, ammonia or sulfur dioxide to destroy the complex salts of caffeine in tea leaves. As the aromatic substances must be retrieved from a fraction of solvent in this process, it is generally not possible to remove all residual solvents.

New processes have been used for the production of black tea without caffeine, which retain the original flavor, that is to say the aromatic content and eliminates previous problems. During the 1970s many patents have been taken to replace the decaffeination process by organic solvents. Only the process of supercritical carbon dioxide is considered the most appropriate because it preserves all the features and keeps the flavor intact. Supercritical carbon dioxide decaffeination is similar to the direct solvent methods. High-pressure vessels are used to circulate the carbon dioxide through a bed of premoistened, tea leave raw material. At high pressure, carbon dioxide has supercritical properties that enhance its solvent properties. Supercritical carbon dioxide has a density like that of a liquid, but its viscosity and diffusivity are similar to those of a gas. These attributes significantly lower its pumping costs. For example, feasibility studies have shown that although the initial cost of the supercritical carbon dioxide plant is higher, this process provides a better income and an increase in gross profit per ton of processed green tea, that the classical process which uses ethyl acetate. The increase in gross profit is primarily due to the excellent quality of both green tea and caffeine produced by the process of supercritical carbon dioxide and the fact that losses are negligible in this process. The applications of supercritical fluid technology in food processing have been carried out mainly using carbon dioxide considered to be an ideal supercritical fluid because it is non-flammable, non-toxic, non-polluting and easy to recover.

The decaffeination process that uses supercritical carbon dioxide as a solvent has been developed by Zosel [3–7] at the Max Planck Institute of Coal Research in Germany. Three ways to make the decaffeination of coffee using compressed carbon dioxide as a solvent have been proposed by Zosel. In the first technique, moistened green coffee beans are contacted with a stream of carbon dioxide in a pressure vessel, at temperatures between 70 and 90 °C and pressures ranging from 16 to 22 MPa. The caffeine diffuses from beans in the carbon dioxide that passes through a washing tower containing water, where the caffeine is separated from carbon dioxide and carbon dioxide saturated water is recycled to the extractor. After 10 h of recycling, the concentration of caffeine in the seeds is reduced to 0.02%. In the second method the extraction conditions are the same as in the first process, but in this case, caffeine which is extracted from carbon dioxide passes through a bed of activated carbon. In the third method, the compressed carbon dioxide at 22 MPa filled a vessel containing a mixture of green coffee and wet granular activated carbon at 90 °C. Under these conditions the caffeine diffuses directly from coffee beans in the carbon pellets through carbon dioxide. Other patents for the decaffeination of coffee with supercritical carbon dioxide were mostly taken in order to improve the elimination of caffeine in continuous processes [8–19].

Several methods for the decaffeination of tea leaves are reported in the literature, most of them concern the decaffeination of moistened black tea. Vitzthum and Hubert extracted caffeine from black tea with supercritical carbon dioxide by removing first the fraction of aromatic tea with dry gas and caffeine with wet gas, and finally the decaffeinated tea is reimpregnated with the aromatic content [20]. Gehrig and Forster obtained first an aroma enriched fraction from the moistened black tea with carbon dioxide from 6 to 15 MPa, in the temperature range 20-70 °C, and added again this fraction into the decaffeinated and dried tea. The decaffeination starts after the aroma fraction was separated by pumping carbon dioxide at a pressure between 15 and 50 MPa and a temperature from 10 to 100 °C, through a bulk moistened tea.

The solvent charged with caffeine is passed over an adsorber or purified by reduction of density [21]. Klima et al. described a process for the decaffeination of tea containing 15 - 50% by weight of water with moist carbon dioxide at 25 - 35 MPa and 50 - 80 °C in a pressure vessel [22]. In the process Schulmeyr [23], the decaffeination of tea takes place with the end-product, which has already all aroma components. Typical extraction conditions when using supercritical carbon dioxide as solvent are pressures between 20 and 30 MPa and temperatures between 10 and 80 °C. Decaffeination is only possible, when the tea leaves are not dry. Therefore the tea was moistened to a water content of 26% (by weight) prior to extraction. The removal of caffeine was done by pressure drop in a separator. The tea typical polyphenols are not soluble under those conditions, and the aroma perception was improved remarkably in comparison to the classical commercial extraction. The effect of co-solvents on the decaffeination of green tea by supercritical carbon dioxide has been studied by Park et al. [24]. The main objective of this work was to provide experimental data on compressed green tea leave raw material, using carbon dioxide in wide ranges of thermodynamic conditions. Surprisingly we found that the contents of caffeine and other ingredients in water brewing were higher with samples preliminarily treated with supercritical carbon dioxide at moderate pressures (7.0–10 MPa) than the one in untreated tea leaf samples. Then we assumed that supercritical carbon dioxide in extractor filled with tea raw material increases the expansion of channels in leaf structure and improves the dissolution of target substances in water phase. The spreading out of leaves with carbon dioxide is a technique that has been employed in the tobacco industry to reduce the bulk density of the tobacco in cigarettes [25, 26]. It has also been used to improve the drying and rehydration properties of fruits and vegetables [27, 28]. The puffing process involves the release or expansion of a gas within a product in order to create an internal cell like structure or to expand and rupture an existing structure. Similar occurrences of imbibitions of polymer materials in supercritical fluid media as well as efficient improvement of cellulose reactivity were found [29]. It should be noticed that so-called liftoff technique applied to cellulose (rapid pressure drop of supercritical fluid medium with submersed sample) [29] proved to facilitate breaking of cross-links in macromolecules of biopolymer and to improve reactivity thereof. Thus, in this paper the authors tackle the physic-chemical problem of the pretreatment of tea raw material by original procedures [30-32], which are performed in order to restructure the tea leaf and they give the conditions to increase the mass-transfer into the liquid phase at the stage of beverage concoction.

2. Original Processing of Commercial Samples of Chinese and Vietnamese Green Teas by Supercritical Carbon Dioxide

In order to increase the mass transfer into liquid phase of the beverage concoction, preliminary procedures for raw tea treatment have been completed : the static treatment which is the conditioning in supercritical carbon dioxide medium [31], CO_2 circulation [30, 32] and multiple decompression in system (feedstock - supercritical carbon dioxide) [30, 32]. The final acceptance for the proposed procedures must be found out in the ways of obtaining an optimal combination of quality of tea leaves in the original beverage, a low cost of the implemented procedures and prospected feedstock savings. Thus, the release of SC-CO_2 within the corresponding procedure is to be carried out with the state parameters, which correspond to the smallest CO_2 dissolving ability with respect to the components of the feedstock on the one hand, and with P and T values, which provide the greatest possible swelling of raw tea on the other hand. Due to the lack of principled differences in properties of Vietnamese and Chinese teas, the authors of the investigation have found it possible to perform measurements on relevant sample in each specific case

2.1. Experimental Study

2.1.1. Materials, Apparatuses and Procedure

Carbon dioxide, of 99.995% purity, was purchased from GOST 8050-85 State Standard (Quality Certificate No. 2052). Vietnamese green tea leaves which were dried "Che Thai Nguyen" were used. Caffeine of analytical grade, with a content of the main component of at least 99.95 wt % was used. Ultra-pure water has been purifying with the device "Millipore Simplicity 185". Two types of supercritical extraction systems were utilized: a badge device (Fig.1) and a circulatory device SCFE-400 (Fig. 2). They are associated to a supercritical fluid chromatograph recorder (Thar Technologies). The spectra are made using a UV/Vis spectrophotometer and a scanning electron microscope EVO 50 XVP (Carl Zeiss) equipped with an energy dispersive spectrometer of 2 nm resolution. The moisture content of green tea leaves of 6% before each experiment was measured by a halogen moisture analyzer HR53-P (Mettler Toledo).

The optimum thermodynamic conditions of the supercritical medium were sought on the one hand to minimize the solubility of feedstock ingredients and secondly to ensure maximum imbibition of tea leaves. For this reason, the solubility of caffeine has been studied in terms of sub and supercritical conditions.

The experiments were conducted in both facilities badge and circulatory devices.

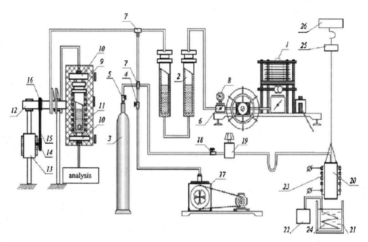

Figure 1. Schematic diagram of a facility for static solubility measurement: in supercritical CO_2 at pressures up to 6.0 MPa and temperatures up to 470 °C. (1) DPG-600 Deadweight pressure gauge; (2) high pressure mercury separator; (3) CO_2 cylinder; (4, 5, 6, 10, 18) high pressure valves; (7) four way connector; (8) reference spring manometer; (9) phase equilibrium vessel; (11) steel ball; (12–16) pumping device; (17) vacuum pump; (19) pressure regulator; (20–24), thermo-compressor; (25) windlass; (26) weighing platform.

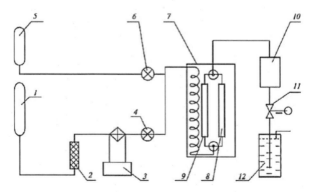

Figure 2. Schematic diagram of a continuous flow solubility measurement facility: (1) CO_2 cylinder; (2) filter-drier; (3) cooler; (4, 6) pumps; (5) co-solvent reservoir; (7) air bath; (8, 9) extractors; (10) ultraviolet detector; (11) pressure regulator; (12) antisolvent reservoir.

In the badge process (Fig.1) green tea leaves are loaded into the high pressure vessel which was afterwards evacuated to end pressure of ~1 Pa. Then, the chamber is filled with carbon dioxide at pressure of the experiment using a thermal compressor. The device temperature control is started. When pressure and temperature are stabilized a stirring device is operated to ensure saturation of the liquid phase and the maintenance of thermodynamic equilibrium. The equilibrium time is defined as the sum of time to stabilize the pressure and time of collection of samples on which the solubility measurements were performed.

Figure 2 illustrates the schematic diagram of a supercritical fluid extraction facility that enables implementation of solubility measurement in dynamic mode. The carbon dioxide contained in a cylinder (1) passes through the filter, (2) filled with silica gel for gas drying. Carbon dioxide is cooled to 268 K, (3) a three-piston pump, (4) delivers a constant flow of gas. If a co-solvent is used (reservoir 5), it is supplied by the dual piston pump, (6) after mixing, the CO_2 and the co-solvent enter into an air flow thermostat, (7) which contains two extractors. Prior to the stabilization of the temperature and pressure within the thermostat, the gas goes in the empty cylinder, (8) and after stabilization of its temperature and pressure, it flows through the extractor, (9) filled with raw material. In operation, the raw ingredients which may be dissolved by the solvent are analyzed in the ultraviolet detector, (10) that registers the composition of the solution.

Optimal conditions for the preliminary treatment of tea leaves must be determined in order to ensure full recovery of raw material. For this reason, the amount of caffeine in tea measured after a 20 min infusion of tea leaves in boiling distilled water was taken as reference for comparative analysis (technique by "Sinteco Sci-Tech Co.). Moreover the rates of caffeine in tea leaves determined by "Sinteco" technique were compared with those obtained by chemical analysis.

2.1.2. Results and Discussion

In figs 3 and 4 are shown the variation of caffeine concentration for different operating modes Figure 3 which illustrates the dependence of caffeine concentration as a function of SC-CO_2 flow rate, enabling to determine equilibrium caffeine concentration in CO_2 by default.

In Figure 4 solubility measurement of caffeine are reported as a function of pressure ranging from 7 to 30 MPa, for nominal temperatures of 308.15 K, 318.15 K and 333.15 K. As shown in this figure, measurements are in good agreement with literature data, obtained at 313.15 K [33].

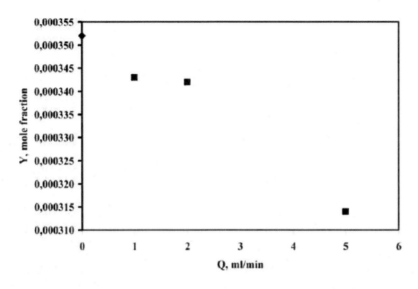

Figure 3. Variation of caffeine concentration in green tea leaves as a function of CO_2 flow rate (T = 308.15 K; P = 30.0 MPa): ♦ static method, ■ dynamic method.

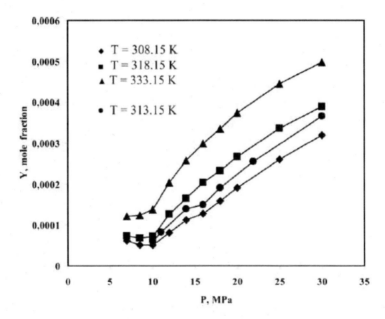

Figure 4. Variation of caffeine solubility in supercritical carbon dioxide as a function of pressure at T=308.15 K, 318.15 K and 333.15 K (present work) and T = 313.15. [33].

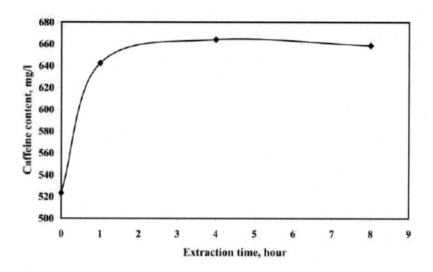

Figure 5. Caffeine content in an aqueous phase of raw tea leaves exposed preliminary to a stream of carbon dioxide at T = 333.15 K and P = 10.0 MPa, for 8 h.

The temperature conditions of the procedure are a compromise between the minimum solubility of tea stock ingredients in supercritical CO_2 and the maximum swallowing of raw material. Fig. 5 shows a considerable increase of extractability in target components in water phase, after pretreatment of tea leaves.

The decreasing of caffeine content observed after 8 h cycle could be explained by partial extraction of caffeine. It should be noted that losses are indeed insignificant. That was corroborated by the level of antisolvent contents through which carbon dioxide is bubbling at the final stage. For instance, the caffeine content in water used as antisolvent varied between 1 and 3 mg.l^{-1} at 10.0 MPa.

Higher values of the pressure of carbon dioxide may facilitate imbibition of tea raw material and thus increase the mass transfer in water brewing. However, it is likely that this will be achieved at the expense of the final product quality, due to increased solubility of the active ingredients in supercritical carbon dioxide. This is confirmed by the experimental results on samples treated at 333.15 K, 30.0 MPa, with a flow rate of CO_2 of 3 ml/min. Fig. 6 shows that the content of caffeine and other ingredients during the brewing was significantly lower with samples of raw material treated than with those of tea leaves untreated.

Utilization Efficiency Improvement ... 149

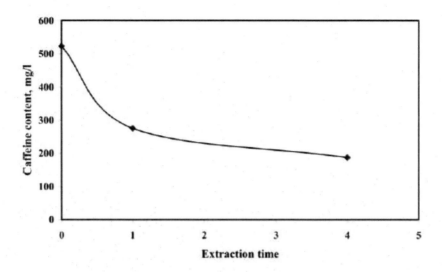

Figure 6. Variation of caffeine content in water brewing of raw tea leaves subjected to a stream of carbon dioxide at T = 333.15 K and P = 30.0 MPa, as a function of extraction time.

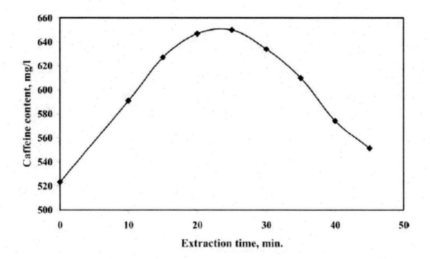

Figure 7. Variation of caffeine content in water brewing of raw tea leaves subjected to a stream of carbon dioxide at T = 333.15 K and P = 40.0 MPa, in terms of extraction time.

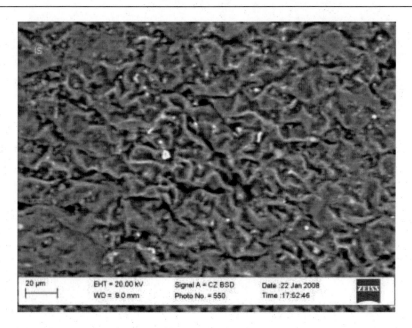

Figure 8. The microphotograph of unprocessed raw tea sample.

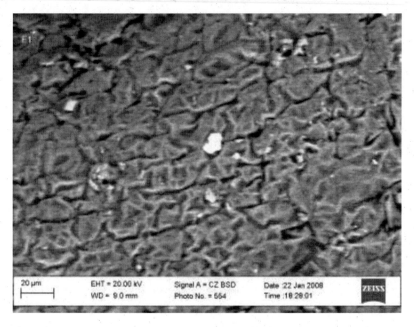

Figure 9. Microphotograph of raw tea sample exposes to a flow of CO_2 at a temperature of 333.15 K and a pressure of 10.0 MPa for 1 h.

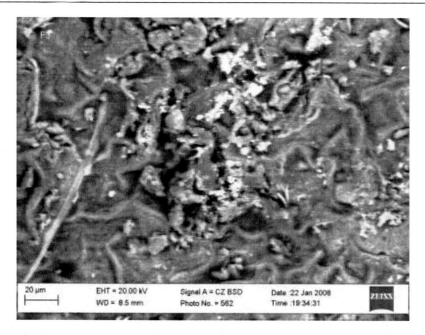

Figure 10. Microphotograph of a raw tea sample exposed previously to a three-stage decompression of 40 min time intervals, from an initial pressure of 40.0 MPa and at a temperature of 333.15 K.

Samples of raw materials of tea leaves were subjected to an initial pressure of carbon dioxide of 40.0 MPa and a temperature of 333.15 K. The system is then decompressed at regular time intervals, after 10, 15, 20, 25, 30, 35, 40, 45 min. After each decompression, the caffeine content in water brewing is measured. Fig. 7 shows the variation of caffeine content after each decompression. It is found that the caffeine content is highest after an exposure time of 25 min. In these experiments, the duration of decompression time is about 10 min.

Information on the structural changes occurring in raw materials during the treatments described above, are illustrated in microphotographs shown in Figs. 8-10. Fig. 8 corresponds to a raw material unprocessed, Fig. 9 to a raw material subjected to flow of carbon dioxide, for one hour, at a temperature of 333.15 K and a pressure of 10 MPa, and Fig. 10 corresponds to a raw material subjected to a temperature of 333.15 K, a pressure of 40.0 MPa and an exposure time of 40 min.

As shown in Fig. 9, the sample which is exposed to the flow of CO_2 at 10 MPa for one hour shows a clear effect of imbibition.

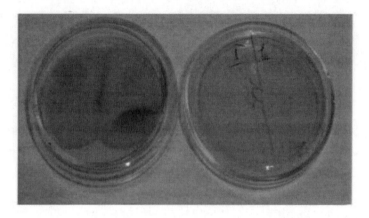

Figure 11. Solutions obtained from bacteriological control of raw tea processed by SC-CO_2 (right). Untreated solution on the left has a heart-shaped outline.

In Fig 10, the sample exposed to pressures of 40 MPa for 40 min, we observe both changes due to imbibition and mechanical modification of the structure, which has the effect of increasing the accessibility of active ingredients in raw materials during water brewing.

Considering again Fig. 7, it shows that the amount of caffeine in treated raw tea depends on two factors. The first is the increase of mass transfer during the water brewing. The second is the elimination of active ingredients during the extraction by supercritical carbon dioxide. The first factor clearly outweighs in the rising part of the curve and the latter shall prevail to the decreasing part.

Bacteriological analysis of samples of tea conducted by the technique of total microbial counts showed the presence of black mold Aspergillus niger in raw materials and the total absence of bacteria after treatment with supercritical carbon dioxide at 313.15 K and 40 MPa (Fig. 11). This is another advantage of the method of processing tea leaves by SC-CO_2.

3. Effect of Processing with Supercritical CO_2 on Composition and Structure of Tea Leaf and Cellulose Resulting from the Analysis of the Solid Phase

Original procedures for the preliminary processing of tea leaves by CO_2 are proposed. These procedures lead to swelling of tea leaves which create structural changes in the solid phase. With the example of caffeine, we show that such structural changes may contribute more efficiently to the use of the biological potential of the tea leaves at the stage of preparing a beverage. In particular, according to the above listed results, conventional caffeine content in tea can be 30 % lower when extracted by the dry process than in the wet process. Thus, the evaluations on the caffeine sample give an idea about the quality safety of the original tea leaf, after the implementation of the procedures discussed above. However, caffeine is far from being the only valuable component of the tea raw material.

Among the most important biological components of tea leaf are plant minerals (PMs). Their composition is very similar to that of minerals present in the fluids of the human body. Minerals contained in plants appeared relatively recently as valuable products, but are already well introduced in the world markets.

The bulk (up to 80 wt %) of the elemental composition of PMs is represented by potassium, chlorine, sodium, and sulfur. Less abundant, but no less important are magnesium, calcium, manganese, iron, copper, phosphorus, selenium, zinc, and even elements such as arsenic, lead, and aluminum. Until recently, many of them were considered toxic, but as it turned out, in weak concentrations and combinations with other substances, they are essential to the human organism.

The minerals with the greater amount in green tea leaves are potassium, calcium, phosphorus, and magnesium. In a lesser amount we have manganese, zinc, copper and iron. Moreover green tea is an extremely good sources of vitamin C, a potent antioxidant. Dietary minerals are very important for our health. Minerals, along with vitamins, are among the five main nutrients essential for the human body. In particular, of the ninety important nutrients, sixty are minerals [34]. It is no accidental that the modern concepts increasingly associate the emergence of diseases with a deficiency of minerals. If in terms of importance to the individual components of food, the XX century could be called the era of vitamins, the XXI century, in this sense, will be the era of minerals

In essence, RMs are inorganic ingredients taken by the plant in the environment and transformed into its organism so that the extent of their assimilation by the human body can reach 98%, whereas untransformed inorganic minerals, are absorbed only in quantities of 3 to 8%.

There are legitimate questions concerning the nature and characteristics of structural changes in tea leaf. What are the changes in the various phases of processing, for example for caffeine within the multiple decompression procedure? It appears that when the supercritical fluid solution of caffeine in carbon dioxide leaves the micro and nanoscale channels of the tea leaf, it entrains a dispersing process that is similar to the RESS process [35-37]. The changes of phase of caffeine crystal produce the changes in kinetics of their dissolution in the aqueous phase [38]. These questions have predetermined the direction of further investigations, the results of which are going to be presented below.

3.1. Experimental Study

3.1.1. Materials, Equipment and Investigation Methods

The preprocessing of tea samples with carbon dioxide was performed on a supercritical fluid extractor installation of circulation type (employing CO_2 circulation mode) equipped with a high-pressure phase equilibrium cell, in which take place the treatment by carbon dioxide and the subsequent decompressions. For the dispersion of the caffeine by RESS method, the laboratory setup RESS-100 by «Thar Technologies» was used (Fig. 12). Microphotographs of the caffeine particles have been made by optical microscope Levenhuk D670T.

The IR spectra of solid samples of cellulose, tea leaf, and caffeine were recorded on a FTIR Perkin Elmer Spectrum 100 series Fourier transform infrared spectrometer, with a spectral resolution of 1.5-2.0 cm^{-1} between 400-4000 cm^{-1}.

The spectra of solid cellulose and tea leaf were recorded using a solid-phase immersion medium (KBr) [39]. The samples were ground in an agate mortar, mixed with powdered KBr in ratios of 1/100 to 1/1000 and pressed in a special mold which provides a mechanical pressure of 8 $ton.cm^{-2}$ under a residual pressure of 2 mmHg.

The elemental composition of the mineral substances in tea leaf was determined using the following standard methods: GOST (State Standard) 30178-96 "Raw materials and food stuffs; atomic absorption method for determination of toxic elements" [40]. GOST 30692-2000 "Fodders, mixed fodders, and animal raw foodstuff; atomic absorption method for determination of copper, lead, zinc, and cadmium" [41]; and GOST 26929-94 "Food raw material and foodstuff; samples preparation; mineralization to determine toxic elements" [42]. The elemental composition of tea leaf was measured on an AAnalyst-200 atomic absorption spectrometer with a double-beam scale optical system and a solid-state semiconductor detector (Perkin Elmer).

The initial materials used in this study have the following gradations and characteristics:

Chinese green tea (Greenfield Flying Dragon; date of manufacture/ packaging, June 2009), carbon dioxide (GOST 8050-85, quality certificate No. 2052; with a CO_2 volume content of 99.995%); caffeine (analytical grade, with a content of the main component of at least 99.95 wt %); and microcrystalline cellulose (Ankir-B grade, Evalar corp.). Water used in the experiments was purified on a Millipore Simplicity 185 water purification system.

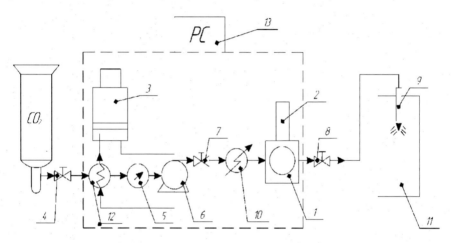

Figure 12. Thar RESS-100 experimental unit: *1*, reactor; *2*, stirrer; *3*, thermostat; *4, 7,* and *8*, valves; *5*, flow meter; *6*, high-pressure pump; *9*, expansion device; *10*, heat exchanger for heating (electrical heater); *11*, expansion chamber; *12*, heat exchanger for cooling; and *13*, PC.

3.1.2. Results and Discussion

The content of minerals in the tea leaves samples after the implementation of the corresponding tea raw materials pretreatment procedures is presented in Figures 13-16.

The increased iron content in the sample treated in the CO_2 circulation mode for 5 h (Fig. 13) is apparently associated with the presence of iron in the devices involved in the processing procedure.

An increase in the temperature and pressure of SC-CO_2 causes no significant change in the elemental composition of tea leaf. However, the cobalt content upon CO_2 circulation (Fig. 14) and decompressions (Fig. 16) decreases. One reason for this reduction may be a high solubility of cobalt in SC-CO$_2$.

To study the effect of SC-CO$_2$ on the structure of tea leaf, we recorded FTIR absorption spectra of tea leaf and cellulose which is one of its components. The IR absorption spectrum of a polymer like cellulose is much complex.

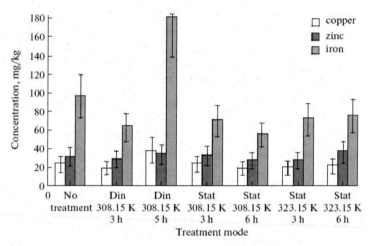

Figure 13. Content of copper, zinc, and iron (mg.kg^{-1}) in a tea leaf before and after the treatment with supercritical CO$_2$ (in quiescent and circulating SC-CO$_2$ at 10.0 MPa); Din. and Stat. mean treatment under dynamic and static conditions.

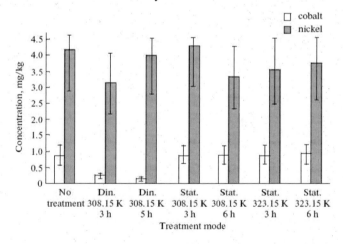

Figure 14. Content of cobalt and nickel (mg.kg$_{-1}$) in a tea leaf before and after treatment with supercritical CO$_2$ (in quiescent and circulating SC-CO$_2$ at 10.0 MPa); Din. and Stat. mean treatment under dynamic and static conditions.

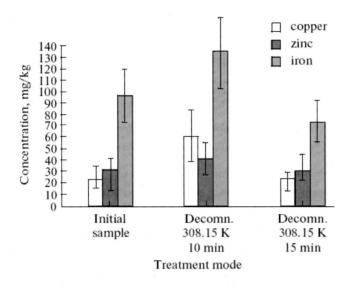

Figure 15. Content of copper, zinc, and iron (mg.kg^{-1}) in tea leaf before and after treatment with supercritical CO_2 (three-fold decompression starting from a pressure of 30.0 MPa).

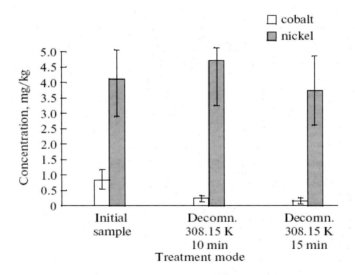

Figure 16. Content of cobalt and nickel (mg.kg^{-1}) in tea leaf before and after treatment with supercritical CO_2 (three steps of decompression stating from a pressure of 30.0 MPa).

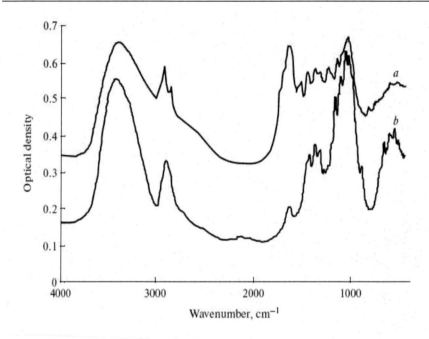

Figure 17. FTIR spectra of (*a*) tea leaf and (*b*) microcrystalline cellulose before SC-CO$_2$ treatment.

Many of observed absorption bands are associated with a large number of different vibrational modes, and cannot be assigned to the vibrations of individual compounds of the cellulose macromolecule.

The intense broad band at 3200-3600 cm^{-1} in the spectra of cellulose and tea leaf belongs to the stretching vibrations of hydroxyl groups O–H involved in hydrogen bonding (Fig. 17).

The intense band at 2800-3000 cm^{-1} belongs to the stretching vibrations of CH$_2$ and CH. The bands of the deformation vibrations of the C–OH and CH groups are located within 1300-1400 cm^{-1}. The strong absorption bands in the region 1000-1200 cm^{-1} are mainly associated with the stretching vibrations of C–O. Due a strong coupling of the vibrations with frequencies in this interval, it is practically impossible to assign the absorption bands observed in the range to particular groups. The bands in the frequency range 700-900 cm^{-1} are attributed to rocking modes of methylene groups, the bending vibrations of C–H bonds and pyran rings. The bands in the region 400-700 cm^{-1} can hardly be assigned. We believe that they largely belong to the bending vibrations of hydroxyl groups and overtones of hydrogen bonds. Absorption at frequencies near 1600 and 1500 cm^{-1} is associated to aromatic impurities (lignin).Moreover, a contribution to the absorption near 1600 cm^{-1} can come from the scissoring vibration of the water molecule. Cellulose has a system of inter- and intra-molecular hydrogen bonds O–H···O. The internal rotations of C–O and C–C bonds give rise to a set of different configurations of cellulose, which differ in the structure of the hydrogen bonds. These configurations play a large role in the biological and physical properties. The number of absorption bands is not an accurate indication of the number of the possible types of hydrogen bonds. In addition a significant part of cellulose material has amorphous domains, which can distort inter-molecular hydrogen bonds.

The absorption bands at 3430 and 1634 cm^{-1} in the spectra of cellulose are formed by a superposition of the vibrational bands of O–H groups which differ in the frequency absorption, the absorption coefficient and an absorption band half-width. These quantities depend on the energy of the hydrogen bond. With increasing hydrogen bond enthalpy, the frequency decreases whereas absorption coefficient and half-width are increasing [43]. The contours of the absorption bands of the stretching vibrations of O–H groups involved in the formation of intra- and intermolecular hydrogen bonds are asymmetric.

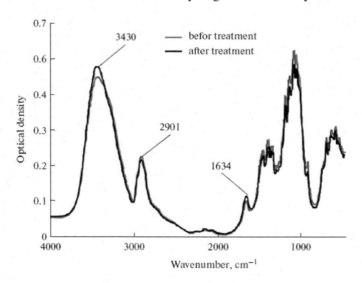

Figure 18. FTIR spectrum of microcrystalline cellulose before and after CO$_2$-treatment (CO$_2$ - circulation).

Figure 18 shows the FTIR spectra of microcrystalline cellulose before and after CO$_2$ treatment perform by CO$_2$ circulation. We examined the relative peak intensities of the absorption bands belonging to the stretching and bending vibrations of groups O–H (3430 and 1634 cm^{-1}) and C–O (~1060 cm^{-1}), more specifically, we estimated the intensity ratios Irel (3430) ≈ $I3430/$ $/I(1060)$ and Irel (1634) = $I(1634)/I(1060)$.

The use of the relative intensities of absorption bands in conjunction with the Beer-Lambert law makes it possible to exclude the influence of the thickness of the tablet and the concentration of cellulose in the KBr matrix on the intensity of the band.

In addition, the analysis of the spectra of pure KBr tablets showed the absence of the background absorption of KBr in the spectral range under consideration.

Treatment by SC-CO$_2$ entrains a restructuring of the framework of intra- and intermolecular hydrogen bonds, an increase in the intensity of the absorption bands at 3430 and 1634 cm^{-1}, and consequently a rise in the number of O–H groups involved in hydrogen bonds. This is probably accompanied by conformational transformations in the molecules of cellulose via rotations about C–C and C–O bonds. As regards the spectrum of tea leaf, the differences in the spectra are most pronounced between 2000-4000 cm^{-1} (Fig. 17). The spectrum of tea leaf exhibits a band at 3390 cm^{-1}, which belongs to the stretching vibrations of O–H groups involved in the formation of intra- and intermolecular hydrogen bonds, while the cellulose spectrum shows a maximum at 3430 cm^{-1}. The half-width of the absorption band at 3430 cm^{-1} is 440 cm^{-1}, and the half-width of the absorption band at 3390 cm^{-1} is ~610 cm^{-1}. The broadening of the latter one being due to a wide and intense wing spreading over a range of wavenumbers smaller than 3390 cm^{-1}. This is indicative of a difference in the networks of hydrogen bonds in cellulose and tea leaf. It turned out that in tea leaf the number of strong hydrogen bonds is larger, as can be seen by the position of peak of the absorption band and the extended wing of the band.

Upon processing tea leaf in SC-CO$_2$, the intensity of the band at 3390 cm^{-1} decreases (Fig. 19). The processing of tea leaves causes a restructuring of the network of intra-and intermolecular hydrogen bonds and reduces the number of O–H···O groups, which absorb near 3390 cm^{-1}. This is probably accompanied by conformational transformations of molecules in tea leaf by means of rotations about C–C and C–O bonds.

The spectrum of crystalline caffeine features a band at 1700 cm^{-1}, which belongs to the stretching vibration of the C=O group; in the amorphous matrix of leaf, it is shifted to 1730 cm^{-1}. Upon processing of tea leaf, the intensity of the 1736 cm^{-1} band decreases (Fig. 20). That means that the processing of tea leaf with SC-CO$_2$ causes a decrease in the content of caffeine in tea leaf.

The amount of caffeine that dissolves in supercritical carbon dioxide and then precipitates like a raw material during the multiple decompression procedure, is greatly inferior to the amount of the caffeine which is soluble in the aqueous phase at the stage of beverage preparation (bypassing the phase of the preliminary dissolution process in SC-CO_2 and deposition from it).

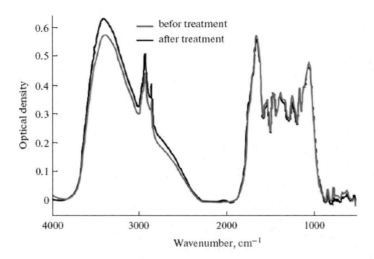

Figure 19. FTIR spectrum of a tea leaf before and after CO_2-treatment (CO_2-circulation).

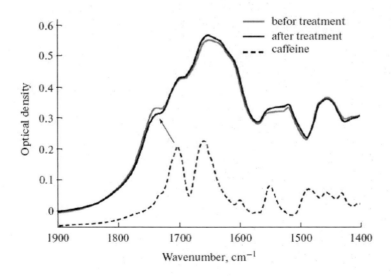

Figure 20. Fragments of FTIR spectra of tea leaf before and after CO_2-treatment (CO_2-circulation) and caffeine.

Table 1. The conditions for RESS-process implementation related to "caffeine - SC-CO$_2$" system

No	P$_{pre}$, MPa	T$_{pre}$, K	D$_{exp.c.}$, micron	T$_{exp}$, K	P$_{exp}$, MPa	τ, min.
1	20	308	200	343	0.1	4
2	38	308	200	343	0.1	4
3*	40	308	750	323	0.1	4

* The sample is taken from the pre-expansion camera after rapid decompression.

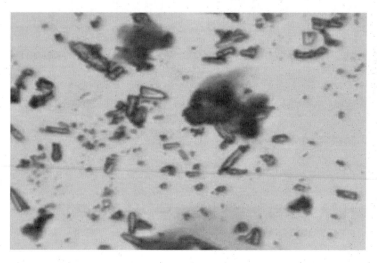

Figure 21. Microphotographs of the initial caffeine particles (average size of large particles: longwise - 98.9 micron, crosswise – 43.2 micron).

However, if we want to model the process as a whole and taking into account the numerous sub-processes, the structural changes, in particular those of caffeine should be studied. The implementation of the RESS method with the caffeine dissolved in supercritical carbon dioxide, considered as a sub-process within the multiple decompression procedure, gives indications on the possible changes in morphology and particle size of caffeine, which should affect the kinetics of dissolution of caffeine in the aqueous phase at the stage of beverage preparing. This information also concerns other components of the tea raw materials which are in some extent soluble in SC-CO$_2$. Table 1 and Figs. 21-24 show the conditions of the implementation of RESS process and its results. The pressure effect on the particles size of caffeine is in a qualitative agreement with the previous results for the same system (caffeine-supercritical carbon dioxide) [35].

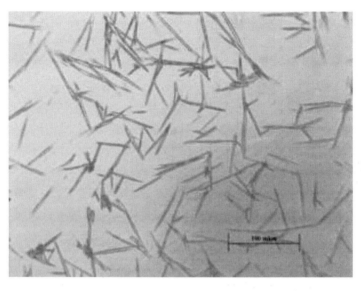
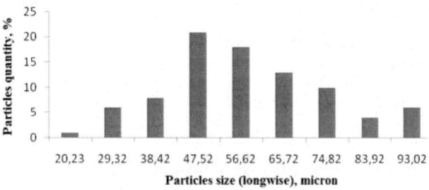
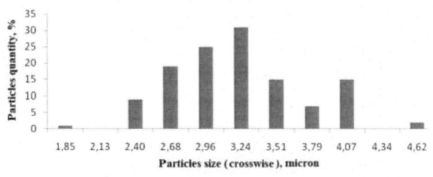

Figure 22. Microphotograph of caffeine particles and their size characteristics for conditions 1 (table 1) of RESS-process implementation.

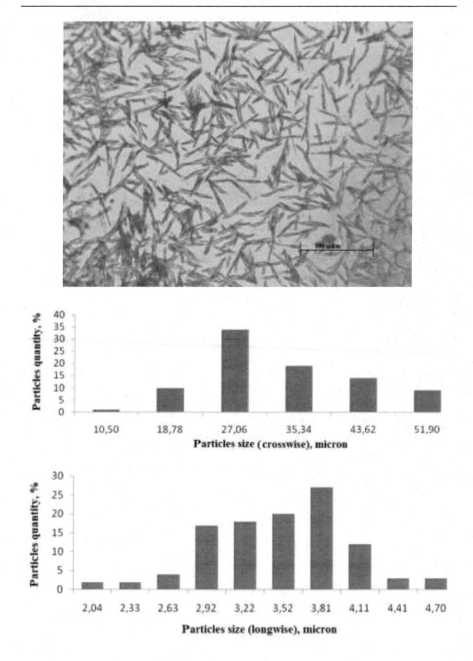

Figure 23. Microphotograph of caffeine particles and their size characteristics for conditions 2 (table 1) of RESS-process implementation.

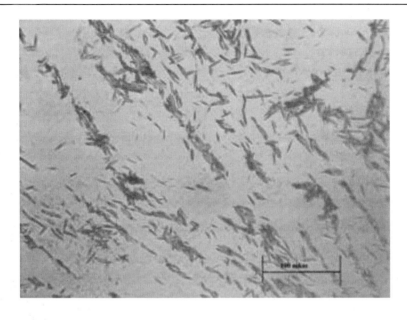

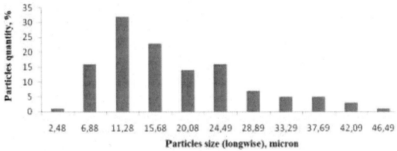

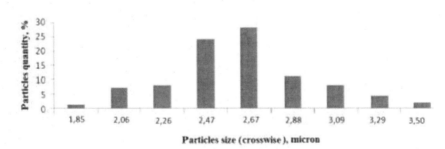

Figure 24. Microphotograph of caffeine particles and their size characteristics for conditions 2 (table 1) of RESS-process implementation (the sample has been taken from the preexpansion camera).

4. Effect of Processing with Supercritical CO2 on Composition and Structure of Tea Leaf and Cellulose Resulting from the Analysis of the Liquid Phase (Beverage)

Taking into account of the analysis results above of the solid phase, and the errors of measurement, we concluded, that in case of preliminary conditioning of tea leaves in SC-CO_2 medium (static process), the content of the minerals in the initial sample of tea is not changed; whereas in the procedure of circulation of SC-CO_2 and multiple decompression, some changes do occur.

However, we have found that the increase of iron content in the tea leaves by applying a dynamic procedure of circulation of SC-CO_2 (Fig. 13) is likely not due to reaction between supercritical carbon dioxide and the tea leaf, but comes from the iron dissolved in the equipment and pipes of the experimental setup. To eliminate the influence of this contribution on the results of this investigation, an analysis of the liquid phase which is presented below has been carried out.

4.1. Experimental Study

4.1.1. Materials, Equipment and Investigation Methods

The elemental composition of tea has been determined using the capillary electrophoresis with the help of «Perkin Elmer» model Prince 560. During the determination of the elemental composition, the following standard methods of analysis of the content have been taken as a basis [44]: GOST R 52930-2008. (Vodka, special vodka and water were used for the concoction. The definition of mass concentration of cations, amines, inorganic anions and organic acids was realized by the method of capillary electrophoresis.

The raw materials used in this study have the following characteristics and gradations:

Chinese green tea by «Greenfield Flying Dragon» (date of manufacture/packing 06.2009), carbon dioxide referenced as GOST 8050-85 (quality certificate number 2052) with a purity of 99.995 %; ultrapure water as a result of purification by Millipore Simplicity 185 apparatus.

4.1.2. Results and Discussion

Table 2 shows the content of the components of tea in beverage samples prepared on the basis of the pre-processed tea leaves following the proposed procedures. The relative error of these quantities is estimated to be ± 11-15%.

We must reminder that chloride is a hydrochloric acid's salt. The barium chloride $BaCl_2$), for example, is used as an insecticide and has intestinal action. The mercuric chloride (II) ($HgCl_2$) or its sublimate is a strongest poison used for disinfection in medicine. The mercuric chloride (I) (Hg_2Cl_2) is used as a laxative in medicine. The sulfate is a salt of sulfuric acid. Oxalates are represented by salts and esters of oxalic acid. The affinity of oxalate to divalent cations is reflected in the ability of formation insoluble precipitates. Inside the organism the oxalates are connected with cations such as Ca2+, Fe2+ and Mg2+, they are forming crystals which irritate the intestinal and kidneys' walls. Whereas oxalates can bind to an important element as calcium, the prolonged consumption of food with an excess of oxalates can be a basis for a wider variety of health problems. The food with a great content of oxalates is not recommended for people with kidney diseases, arthagra or rheumatoid arthritis. Calcium oxalate crystals (kidney stone) clog the kidney ducts. It is believed that up to 80% of kidney stones are presented, namely, by calcium oxalate. Malates mean the salts and anions of malic acid and citrates are represented by salts and esters of citric acid.

In this case, but only as a first approximation, taking into account the errors of measurements, the procedure of static processing of raw materials conditioning in SC-CO_2 medium, can be regarded as an approach that does not modify the content in minerals, including the salts and the esters in the tea beverage, (Figs. 25-28).

It is obvious that the errors of measurement influence singularly the results, they are always present, in particular, in the form of obvious trends, in particular, for all variations of working conditions of static processing (2-9 in table 2). The oxalates content increases up to a maximum of about 9%. The malate content is reduced to a maximum of ~ 15%. The citrates content increases to a maximum of ~ 40% (!!!). The sodium content in all cases exceeds the value for the original raw materials. The increasing of potassium content is inherent to the large majority of conditions under static processing. Moreover, if an increase of oxalates, citrates, and other components is quite easily understood by the fact of swelling of the tea leaf with a corresponding increase in accessibility of target component to the aqueous phase. Nevertheless, in this case, the decreasing of the malate content is difficult to understand and requires further analysis and relevant experiment.

Table 2. The content of tea raw components in beverage samples prepared on the basis of the pre-processed (within the proposed procedures) tea leaves

Sample No.	Processing conditions	Pressure, MPa	Temperature, °C	Processing duration, h	Components concentration mg/kg									
					Chlorides	Sulphates	Oxalates	Malates	Citrates	K	Ca	Na	Mg	Mn
1	Without processing	1			7,25	17,93	76,04	26,34	11,93	186,00	4,81	0,00	11,94	54,96
2	Static	10	35	3,00	6,63	17,15	76,05	22,60	14,26	181,42	4,68	0,34	11,35	52,28
3	Static	10	35	5,00	6,79	17,40	77,00	22,94	13,63	178,72	4,66	1,10	11,16	50,45
4	Static	10	50	3,00	7,27	18,32	78,44	24,54	15,54	189,29	4,96	0,50	11,59	53,22
5	Static	10	50	6,00	7,31	18,97	82,41	23,39	16,69	197,56	5,28	1,35	12,51	57,24
6	Static	20	35	3,00	7,08	17,24	78,29	23,50	14,66	188,92	4,17	0,83	11,66	55,78
7	Static	20	35	6,00	6,45	16,12	76,80	23,83	14,85	183,55	4,64	1,41	11,88	53,77
8	Static	20	50	3,00	6,99	18,07	76,27	24,53	15,86	192,90	4,16	1,47	11,58	51,78
9	Static	20	50	6,00	7,06	17,52	80,64	24,65	15,73	195,48	5,20	1,49	12,65	62,05
10	Decomp.	30	35	0,17	6,88	17,78	73,87	22,76	13,82	182,45	4,45	0,79	11,17	51,12
11	Decomp.	30	35	0,25	7,11	19,64	76,31	23,62	14,47	184,10	4,66	0,85	11,53	57,01
12	Dynamic	10	35	3,00	7,44	16,74	73,77	22,13	11,03	208,86	5,07	0,34	14,21	61,04
13	Dynamic	10	35	5,00	6,25	14,25	65,92	18,35	12,10	173,95	4,61	0,29	11,07	49,79

Utilization Efficiency Improvement ... 169

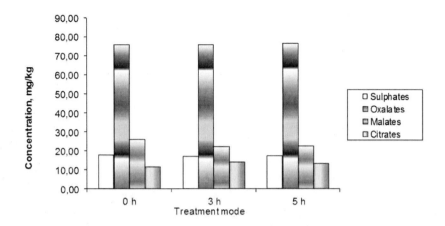

Figure 25. Content of sulphates, oxalates, malates and citrates (mg.kg^{-1}) in a tea beverage, obtained on tea leaves recovered after static processing (conditioning in supercritical carbon dioxide medium at P=10.0 MPa and T=308 K).

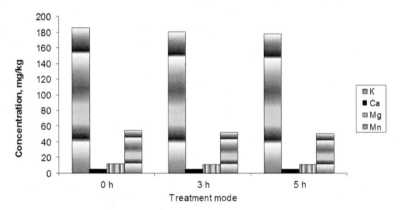

Figure 26. The content of micro and macro-elements (mg.kg^{-1}) in a tea beverage, obtained on tea leaves recovered after static processing (conditioning in supercritical carbon dioxide medium at P=10.0 MPa and T=308 K).

Some obvious trends are observed in the frames of analysis by iso-lines (P, T, τ). They show the presence of interactive links between structural changes in a tea leaf and changes in extractability of the target components in the tea beverage concoction. In particular, the increase in temperature from 35 °C to 50 °C of the following conditions: P/ τ = 10 MPa / 3:00; P / τ = 10 MPa / 5:00; P / τ = 20 MPa / 6:00 is accompanied by an increase in content of all the components listed above of tea raw material.

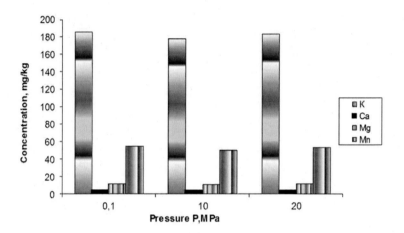

Figure 27. The content of micro and macro-elements (mg.kg^{-1}) in a tea beverage, obtained on tea leaves recovered after static processing (conditioning in supercritical carbon dioxide medium for 3 hours at T=308 K).

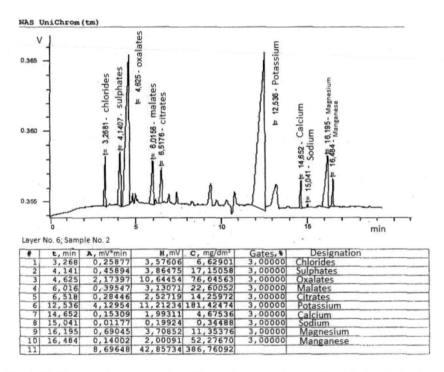

Figure 28. Content chromatography of the tea beverage (sample 2, table 2), obtained on tea leaves recovered after static processing (conditioning in supercritical carbon dioxide medium for 3 hours at P=10 MPa and T=308 K).

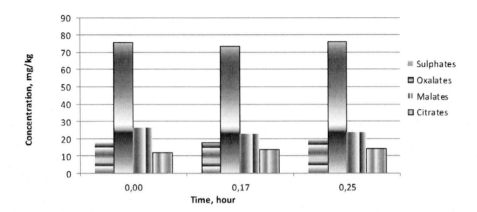

Figure 29. The content of sulphates, oxalates, malates and citrates (mg.kg^{-1}) in a tea beverage, obtained on tea leaves recovered after processing, following the multiple decompression method at P=30.0 MPa and T=308 K.

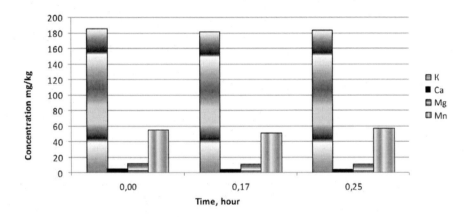

Figure 30. The content of minerals (mg.kg^{-1}) in a tea beverage, obtained on tea leaves recovered after processing, following the multiple decompression method at P=30.0 MPa and T=308 K.

The increase in time of the pretreatment procedure from 3 to 6 hours leads to an increase in content of the large majority of minerals and salts tested, but only when the treatment was carried out at 50 °C. In the processing of tea leaves at temperature 35 °C, this trend has not been established.

The effect of the method of decompression on minerals and salts in the tea beverage (Figs. 29 -30) during the feedstock pretreatment (Samples 10-11 in table 2) is systematic and the variations of forms are obvious.

In particular, the sample 10 (Table 2), treated by triple-decompression after a 10 minute conditioning, is characterized by a large decrease of the majority of minerals and salts.

On the other hand, the increase of the time of conditioning up to 15 minutes (sample 11 in Table 2) is accompanied by an increase of the content of all components in the tea beverage. Thus, we are in presence of at least two trends, entraining structural changes in a tea leaf. In one case, they determine the reduction of extractability, and in the other case they contribute to its increase.

The pretreatment of raw tea in dynamic mode (SC-CO_2 - circulation) significantly affects the final content of minerals and salts in tea (Figs. 31-32, table 3, 4). Changes are obvious and definitely systematic.

If It is logical to assume that the swelling of the tea leaves in the SC-CO_2, associated with increased extractability in aqueous phase, in the process flow of SC-CO_2, is responsible for the increase in the content of minerals (K, Ca, Na, Mg, Mn), in the tea-based beverage prepared with sample 12 (Table 2), however, in the case of Sample 13 (Table 2), the reducing of the content of the majority of the minerals is due to the opposite effect.

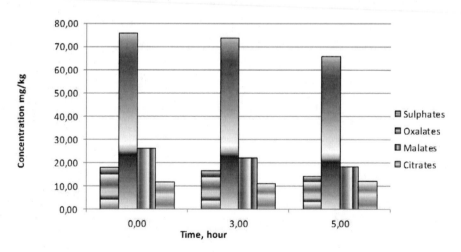

Figure 31. The content of sulphates, oxalates, malates and citrates (mg.kg^{-1}) in a tea beverage, obtained on tea leaves recovered after the pretreatment in dynamic mode at P=10.0 MPa and T=308 K.

Table 3. The change in content of salts and esters in tea beverage as a result of pretreatment of the raw materials in a dynamic mode

Sample No (table 2)	Duration of the procedure, hour	Chlorides	Sulphates	Oxalates	Malates	Citrates
1	0	0%	0%	0%	0%	0%
12	3	2%	-7%	-3%	-19%	-8%
13	5	-14%	-26%	-15%	-44%	1%

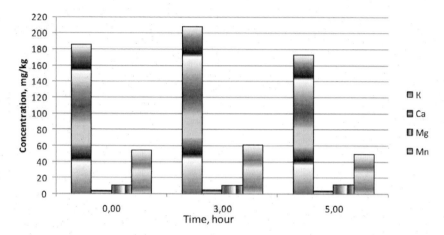

Figure 32. The content of minerals (mg.l^{-1}) in a tea beverage, obtained on tea leaves recovered after the treatment in a dynamic mode (SC-CO$_2$ circulation) at P=10 MPa and T=308 K.

Table 4. The change in content of minerals in tea beverage as a result of pretreatment of the raw materials in a dynamic mode

Sample No (table 2)	Duration of the procedure, hour	K	Ca	Mg	Mn
1	0	0%	0%	0%	0%
12	3	11%	5%	16%	10%
13	5	-7%	-4%	-8%	-10%

In conclusion, with the increase of extractability of caffeine of a tea leaf, into the aqueous phase of brewing beverage, resulting of pretreatment in supercritical carbon dioxide, we noticed that the selection of appropriate handlings to extract other groups of target components (Fig. 33) may contribute to a more efficient knowledge of natural potential of biological materials in the traditional tea concoction.

In this work, we performed the analysis of components content, including caffeine, on samples obtained after 20 minutes brewing of tea leaves in boiling distilled water (method of scientific and technological campaign «SINTECO») [30, 32].

Of course, the beverage brewing conditions may be different. In particular, in [45, 46] the authors have conducted a detailed kinetics study for the release of antioxidants, caffeine, and one of the catechins representative into aqueous phase when beverage brewing at different temperatures of the aqueous phase for the green and black teas.

It is also important to say that, according to the results presented in [47], the SC-CO_2- treatment of raw tea has no negative effect on the activity of antioxidants and other organic active components of a tea leaf.

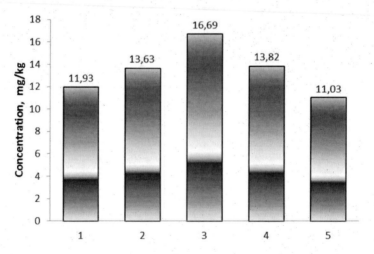

Figure 33. The content of citrates (mg.kg^{-1}) in a tea beverage, obtained on tea leaves recovered after pretreatment procedures discussed above (static, decompression and dynamic) in supercritical carbon dioxide medium. (1) – initial sample; (2) – static mode (10.0 MPa, 308 K, 5 hours); (3) - static mode (10.0 MPa, 323K, 6 hours); (4) – decompression (30.0 MPa, 308 K, 0.17 hour); (5) – dynamic mode (10.0 MPa, 308 K, 3 hours)).

5. THERMAL EFFECT OF CAFFEINE DISSOLVED IN SUPERCRITICAL CARBON DIOXIDE

On the example of tea leaf pretreatment with supercritical carbon dioxide a significant (30%) increase in extractability of natural material's physiologically active substances (PASNM) during the subsequent liquid extraction.

The tea leaf contains cellulose, amino acids etc. Cellulose is a natural polymer whose structure is saturated with PASNM. During the interaction of polymeric material with sub- or supercritical fluid media (SCF) their swelling occurs as a rule, whereby the molecular structure, local dynamics and free volume of these polymers may undergo very significant changes. Thus, the molecular dynamics of polymers is of a great theoretical and practical interest, because the types of molecular motion, which are presented in polymer, strongly affect its mechanical, thermal, dielectric and diffusion properties. In particular, local dynamics determines the secondary relaxation transitions in glassy polymers. Molecular mobility of the polymer is closely related to its free volume. Thermal effects occurring at the stage of the pretreatment of the plant in supercritical carbon dioxide, due to possible dissolving processes of its components into SCF, play a significant role for the conservation of natural qualities of valuable components of natural plant materials as well as for the final extraction of PASNM. The importance of this is primarily related to the fact that the thermal effect supplied from the outside in the process may lead to higher values of temperature outside the limits of stability of PASNM.

The measurements of enthalpy of mixing were mainly concentrated on gas-liquid systems, SCF - liquid such as CO_2-H_2O [48], H_2S-H_2O [49], and CO_2 - methyl diethanolamines aqueous solutions [50]. There is almost no experimental study of enthalpy of mixing for (gas - solid) system, at the exception of the one reported in [51], where the measured enthalpy of mixing is reported for the system (caffeine - CO_2). Excess thermodynamic functions can be derived from phase equilibrium data [52-53] or calculated from equations of state [54-56].However, the differentiation of P-V-T data leads to significant errors in the results of calorimetric measurements. The reliability of redundant functions calculated using different models can be confirmed by their agreement with the direct measurements of these functions.

The result of measurements of thermal effects occurring during the treatment of the main components of tea (caffeine, cellulose, tea leaf) in supercritical carbon dioxide (SC-CO_2) are presented.

5.1. Experimental Study

The investigation of the thermal effects of dissolution of the main tea components in supercritical carbon dioxide has been carried out with an experimental equipment implemented in a heat-conducting calorimeter [57] (Fig. 1). It is equipped with an automatic data recorder and processing [58]. The design of the basic units of this equipment is described in details in [58-61].

5.1.1. Materials, Equipment and Investigation Methods

The initial materials, used in the framework of this investigation have the following gradations and characteristics: the carbon dioxide referred as GOST 8050-85 (quality certificate number 2052) has a purity of 99.995 %; AR grade caffeine with a purity of 99.95% in the target component; microcrystalline cellulose of Ankir-B from Evalar company; ultrapure water was purify using the Millipore Simplicity 185 device.

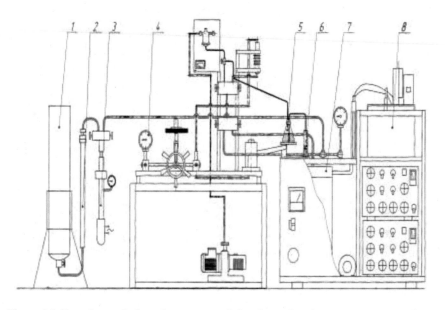

Figure 34. Experimental plant: 1 – gas vessel; 2 – dryer; 3 – thermo-compressor; 4 – deadweight pressure gage; 5, 6 – flow meter; 7 – micro-calorimeter; 8 – thermostating system.

The determination of CO_2 concentration in binary mixture has been carried out using the weighing method. The weigh was measured using the analytical scales VLA-200 and the electronic scales Metter PM 600.

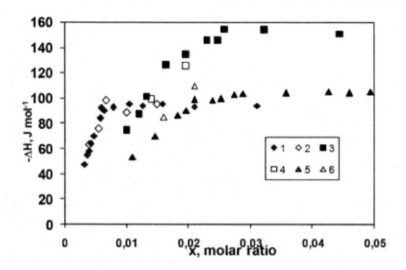

Figure 35. Results of the measurements of enthalpy of dissolution for the binary system (CO_2-H_2O): at P=2 MPa : (1)-[48];(2)-author; at P=10.5 MPa : (3)-[48], (4)-author; at P=20.8 MPa :(5)-[48], (6)-author.

For the investigation of thermal effects, a heat conducting calorimeter was used. The principle of the measuring method is to determine the heat flow rate, which comes from the cell and acts on the thermoelectric battery, located in micro-calorimetric element. The heat flow in the cell mentioned above is the sum of the heat, which is generated or absorbed by the compounds in the cell during the processes of mixing and dissolution as well as compression and thermal expansion. The formula used for the calculation of the thermal effect of mixing (dissolution) ΔH has the following form [48]:

$$\Delta H = \frac{F}{\Sigma \cdot \eta}, \qquad (1)$$

where ΔH is the mixing heat of dissolution (in J.mol-1) and F the thermogram area of the gas or mixture (in V.sec) ; η is the mole fraction of the solute substance or gas (in mole) and Σ the sensibility of the thermo-battery (in μV.mW-1). Calibration measurements of the mixing enthalpy have been carried out with the binary system (CO_2-H_2O), for which there is credible experimental data [45]. The reliability of the thermal effects is confirmed by the measurements of dissolution enthalpy for the binary system (CO_2-H_2O). The deviation of our results from the literature does not exceed 6.9%. The confidence interval of the total error (0.95) related to the dissolution of heat do not exceed ± 3%.

Methodology for Conducting the Experiments

The measurements of thermal effects of dissolution for gas-solid or liquid-solid systems are carried out in the cell provided with a microvalve described in [58, 61].

The measuring cell is carefully cleaned, then weighed using analytical scales VLTE-150 (accuracy class II), and filled with the investigated substance using the free-shoveling method. The cell is weighed again, set up inside the micro-calorimeter and connected to the pressure generating system. Then the operating pressure is produced by the thermo-compressor.

Measurements are taken when the stationary state is reached. The time for reaching the stationary state depends on temperature of the experiment and varies from 2 to 6 hours. Before the starting of measurements the experimental settings are fixed in the controlling program and the experimental zero is set. If the zero drift does not exceed 10-20 mV in 40 minutes, the program starts. Then the cell containing the test substance is supplied with the gas through the high pressure valve, and the saturation of the sample takes place. The saturation process occurs at a constant pressure and is accompanied by a change in temperature, which is recorded by the differential thermo-battery enclosed into the measuring circuit. The differential thermocouples amplified the loop of the error signal which comes from the bridge circuit; it is converted and transferred to the computer by periodic questioning of tracking ADC. Each value is the average of 10 measurements. During the experiment, the accumulation of measurement points takes place; these points are recorded in a data file. The temperature of the fluid in the cell is controlled by a thermo-battery. When the measurements are finished, the program proceeds to the processing of the data. The program allows the calculation of the area of the thermogram corresponding to the heat flow from the cell. All the data are displayed on the monitor in a convenient form for the operator. Then, after the completion of the measurements, the depressurizing is carried out and the thermal processes occurring are registered, there are followed by the calculation of these quantities. The amount of dissolved gas is determined by the gravimetric method in the following way. As soon as the investigated substance is filled or poured in a cell with the same amount as in the main experiment, it is connected to the gas filling system. Then the cell is inserted in a special unit, which is located in the thermostat, so the saturation is carried out as described earlier during the same time as for the determination of thermal effects of the previous experiment. Next, the cell is closed, disconnected from the pressure system and the cell contents are weighed. Then, the gas is discharged from the cell and the cell is closed again and weighed. The gas discharge is carried out at the temperature of the experiment.

5.1.2. Results and Discussion

The results of measurements of the enthalpy of dissolution are shown in Figs.36-40. Different types of behavior were observed when the substances under investigation are dissolved in supercritical carbon dioxide.

The greatest changes in the variation of enthalpy as a function of temperature, take place in the pressure range 8-20 MPa. With the increase of temperature, the absolute value of the thermal effect of mixing decreases, the factor, also is decreasing. Compared to the mixture of (caffeine - $SC-CO_2$), the mixture of (cellulose - $SC-CO_2$) has a lower value (figure 38): This is due to different macromolecular types of structures of caffeine [62] and cellulose [63-67]. Cellulose is a biopolymer with an average molecular weight of 100000-1500000, exceeding the molecular weight of caffeine (MW = 194.2). The units of the macromolecule of cellulose are arranged in parallel, the recurring unit of the macromolecule of cellulose contains groups able to form hydrogen bonds. The heat of dissolution of cellulose in $SC-CO_2$ is comparable to that of cellulose in water ~-3.5 kJ/mole, at T = 303 K [68, 69].

Figure 39 shows a comparison of the heat of dissolution of the main components of a tea leaf in $SC-CO_2$, which confirms that caffeine and cellulose have almost identical values of enthalpy.

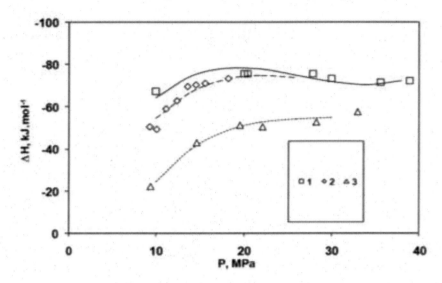

Figure 36. Heat of dissolution of caffeine in SC-CO$_2$ as a function of pressure at different temperatures: 1 – 308 K; 2 – 323 K; 3 – 343 K.

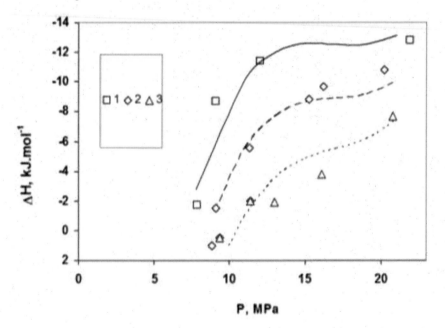

Figure 37. Heat of dissolution of cellulose in SC-CO$_2$ as a function of pressure at different temperatures: 1 – 308 K; 2 – 323 K; 3 – 348 K.

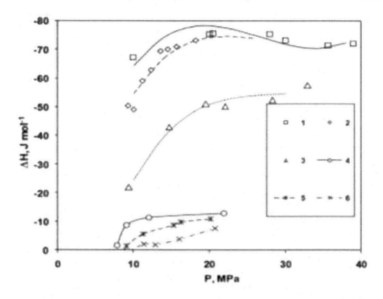

Figure 38. Enthalpy of dissolution (ΔH) of caffeine and cellulose in SC-CO$_2$ at different temperatures as a function of pressure: 1 – caffeine (T=308 K); 2 – caffeine (T=323 K); 3 — caffeine (T=343 K); 4 – cellulose (T=308 K); 5 – cellulose (T=323 K); 6 – cellulose (T=343 K).

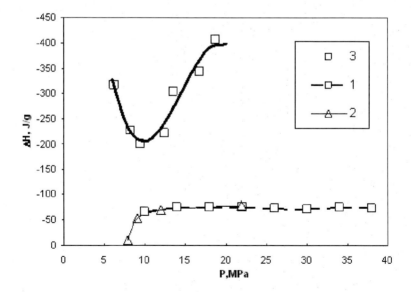

Figure 39. Enthalpy of dissolution (ΔH) of tea leaf components in SC-CO$_2$: 1 – caffeine (T=308 K); 2 – cellulose (T=308 K); 3 – tea leaf (T=304,4 K).

6. Thermodynamic Properties of Binary and Ternary Mixtures Containing Cellulose, Caffeine, Carbon Dioxide and Water, in Supercritical Fluid Conditions

The thermo-physical properties of the individual compounds and binary systems having tea leaves as one of their component have been studied in details [32, 33, 51, 66, 68-87], especially CO_2 [70, 71]. The heat capacity of pure caffeine was measured by various authors [72-74, 76-79]. However, the deviation of the experimental data exceeds the total measurement error which can be possibly associated with purity of the sample. For caffeine used in the study, heat capacity measurements have been carried out in the temperature range of $T = 323K \div 560K$.

The literature contains information about the heat capacity of system of (caffeine-carbon dioxide) [81] at a single concentration and high pressures and the heat capacity of caffeine in aqueous solutions [82-84]. There is no density data for the (caffeine - SC-CO_2) system, although data are available for the aqueous solutions of caffeine [82, 84].

6.1. Experimental Study

6.1.1. Materials, Equipment and Investigation Methods

The study of the heat capacity of caffeine was performed with an automatic apparatus developed as a scanning calorimeter labeled ITS-400 [88, 89].

The working formula of the method is given by:

$$c_P(P, T) = c_P''(T) \cdot \frac{m''}{m} \cdot \frac{\tau - \tau_0}{\tau'' - \tau_0} \cdot, \tag{2}$$

where $C_P(P, T)$, $C_P''(T)$ are isobaric heat capacities of the investigated sample at pressure P, temperature T and reference sample at pressure P_0 and temperature T, (in $J.kg^{-1}.K^{-1}$)); m and m'' are masses of sample and reference substance, (in kg); τ and τ'' are delay times of the measuring thermocouples respectively for the investigated and reference samples (in sec); τ_0 is delay time of the measuring thermocouples for the empty measuring cell (in sec).

To test the efficiency of the experimental set up, measurements were performed to determine the heat capacity of stearic acid (chemically pure grade) at atmospheric pressure and the heat capacity of n-butyl alcohol (n_D^{20} = 1.3995, ρ^{25} = 809.5 kg/m^3) at pressure up to 30 MPa.

The results of these measurements and their comparison with literature data are presented in Figure 40. The deviations of C$_P$ of stearic acid up to the melting point [90] do not exceed 2.1 % compared to the literature data, but C$_P$ of n- butyl alcohol is systematically underestimated by 2% [91]. The latent heat of liquid-crystal, calculated from the heat capacity value of stearic acid was found to be 61.6 kJ.mol^{-1}.K^{-1}, the deviation from the literature data does not exceed 0.7 % The confidence interval of the total measurement error of heat capacity (0.95) does not exceed ± 2%. The determination of the density was conducted by the pycnometric method. The weighing has been carried on with the help of analytical scales model VLA-200, associated with an electronic scale Metter PM 600. The experiment has been set up in an ultra-thermostat U-10, which has an accuracy of regulation of ± 0.02 °K

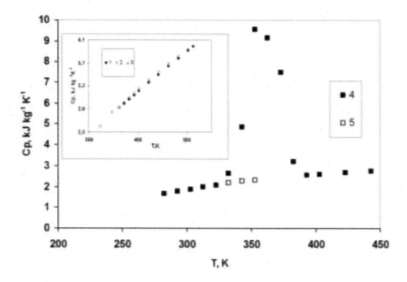

Figure 40. Results of control measurements of Cp and comparison with the literature data for (a): *n*-butyl alcohol (1–author, 2–[91-92]); (b) stearic acid (3–author, 4–[90]).

For the investigation of heat capacity of binary mixture and thermal phenomena in ternary mixture, the heat-conducting calorimeter has been used [58, 61].

The principle of the measuring method is to determine the heat flow rate, which comes from the cell and acts on the thermoelectric battery, located in the micro-calorimetric element. The heat flow in the cell is measured with differential thermocouples.

The densities of binary and ternary mixtures are determined by the gravimetric method in a cell at constant volume provided with a microvalve. The same amount of the investigated substance is poured in a cell as in the main experiment, and the cell is connected to the gas filling system. Then the cell is inserted in a special device, which is located in the thermostat, so the saturation is carried out as described earlier during the same time as for the determination of thermal effects.

Next, the cell is closed, disconnected from the pressure system and the cell content is weighed. Then, the gas is discharged from the cell and again the cell is closed and weighed. The discharge of gas is carried out at the temperature of the experiment.

6.1.2. Results and Discussion

The measurement results of the specific heat of pure caffeine, binary mixture caffeine - SC-CO_2 and its density and ternary mixture caffeine - SC-CO_2 are presented in Figures 41-43.

The deviations of pure caffeine's heat capacity values, obtained by the authors do not exceed 4% (T = 323K), comparing to [78, 79] (Figure 41). Cp values [73] overrate our data and [78, 79] by 6% at T = 373 K. The disagreement with [76] is 4.6% at T = 503K. In the temperature range of T=373-473K deviation from the data [76] do not exceed 2%. Generally deviations from the literature data are within the total measurement error.

Measurements of the heat capacity and density of the binary mixture of (caffeine − SC-CO_2) have been carried out at sub and supercritical pressures. As it can be seen from Fig.42, the heat capacity of this system is inferior to C_P of pure CO_2. The largest deviations are typical for the isotherm of T = 308 K close to critical temperature. With the increase of pressure and temperature, the heat capacity moves towards C_P of pure CO_2.

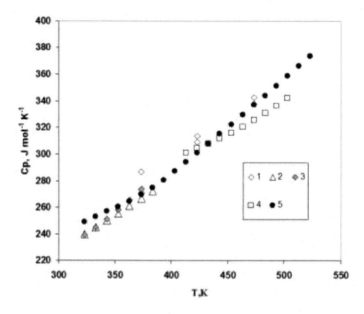

Figure 41. Variation of the heat capacity of caffeine as a function of temperature: 1 – [72]; 2 – [77]; 3 – [75]; 4 – [78]; 5 – author.

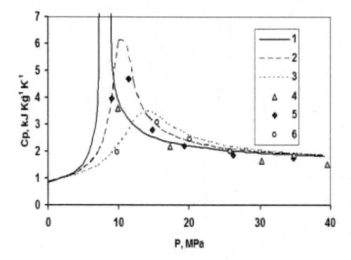

Figure 42. Heat capacity of (caffeine – SC-CO_2) systems as a function of pressure (SC-CO_2 [70]): 1- (SC-CO_2) T = 308 K; 2 – (SC-CO_2) T = 323 K; 3 – (SC-CO_2) T = 343 K; (caffeine -SC-CO_2) [79]; 4 –T = 308 K; 5 –T = 323 K; 6 –T = 343K.

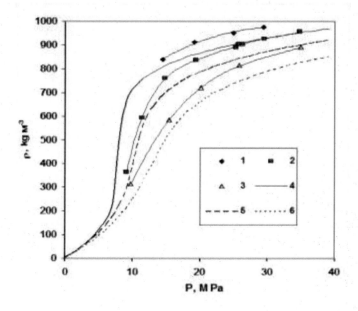

Figure 43. Density of (caffeine – SC-CO$_2$) as a function of pressure: (a) (caffeine – SC-CO$_2$) 1 –T = 308 K; 2 –T = 323 K; 3 –T = 343 K; (b) (SC-CO$_2$) [70]: 4 –T = 308 K; 5 –T = 323K; 6 – T = 343 K.

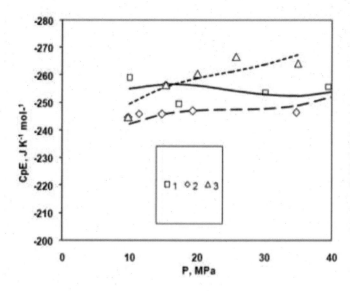

Figure 44. Excess heat capacity of the system (caffeine – SC-CO$_2$) as a function of pressure: 1 –T = 308 K; 2 – T = 323K; 3 – T = 3 43K.

The density of the system (caffeine - SC-CO$_2$) (Fig. 43) is somewhat greater than the density of pure CO$_2$. The variations of the density as a function of temperature and pressure of the system (caffeine - SC-CO$_2$) are similar to those of pure CO$_2$.

The results of Cp measurement for caffeine - SC-CO$_2$ mixture were converted to excessive heat capacity using the following formula:

$$c_p^E = Cp - (Cp_{caff} + Cp_{co_2} N_{CO_2}) \quad (3)$$

where is the excess heat capacity (in J.mol-1.K-1)); Cp is the heat capacity of the mixture (in J.mol^{-1}.K^{-1}); and are the heat capacities of caffeine and SC-CO$_2$ (in J.mol-1.K-1); is the mole fraction of CO$_2$ in the mixture. The calculations were performed using Cp_{CO_2} data [70] and the results of the combined processing of [78, 79] with the author's data.

The obtained data were recalculated by the formula:

$$c_p^E = \left(\frac{\partial h^E}{\partial T}\right)_{p,n_k} = \left(\frac{\partial \Delta h^m}{\partial T}\right)_{p,n_k} \quad (4)$$

into an excessive enthalpy ΔH (figure 45).

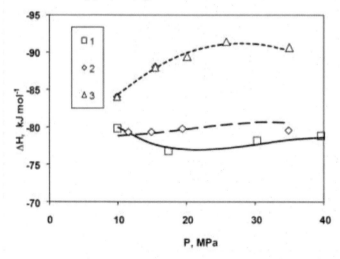

Figure 45. Enthalpy of dissolution (ΔH) of caffeine in SC-CO$_2$ at different temperatures as a function of pressure, calculation: 1 – T = 308 K; 2 –T = 323 K; 3 – T = 343K.

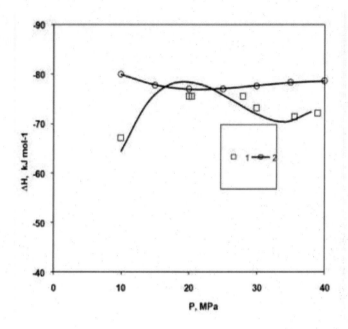

Figure 46. Comparison of the enthalpy of dissolution (ΔH) of caffeine in SC-CO$_2$ at temperature T = 308K: 1 – experiment; 2 - calculation.

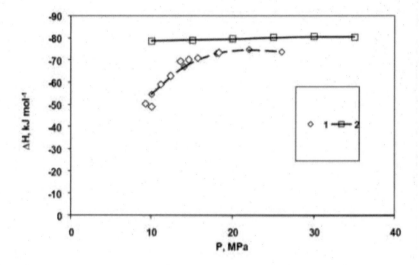

Figure 47. Comparison of the enthalpy of dissolution (ΔH) of caffeine in SC-CO$_2$ at temperature T = 323K: 1 – experiment; 2 - calculation.

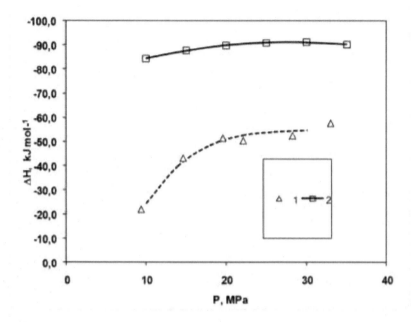

Figure 48. Comparison of the enthalpy of dissolution (ΔH) of caffeine in SC-CO$_2$ at temperature T = 343 K: 1 – experiment; 2 - calculation.

The comparison of the calculated and experimental results (Figs.46-48) shows a qualitative agreement. The largest deviations are observed in the pressure range 10 to 20 MPa..

However, the best agreement is obtained for the isotherms 308 K and 323 K, in the pressure range 15 to 25 MPa.

The excess enthalpy can also be evaluated from solubility data. Thus, in [51], the calculation of excess enthalpy of the mixture (SC-CO$_2$-caffeine) was carried out using a thermodynamic model. With this model and the thermodynamic relations which express the equality of fugacity for solid and liquid phases $f_1^S = f_2^F$, the following correlations to determine the enthalpy from the solubility data were obtained by the authors [51]:

$$H_2^E = R \cdot \left[\frac{\partial \ln \varphi_2}{\partial (1/T)} \right]_P \quad (5)$$

where the logarithm of the fugacity coefficient is evaluated by the formula:

$$\ln \varphi_2 = \frac{V_2^S}{RT} \cdot P - \ln\left(y_2 \cdot \frac{P}{P_0}\right) \qquad (6)$$

where is the coefficient of fugacity of caffeine; is the molar volume of caffeine; is the solubility of caffeine; is the vapor pressure of pure caffeine; P and T are the pressure and the temperature.

The enthalpy values ΔH have been calculated using literature data for [32-33, 51], [51, 72, 75, and 81] and [51, 74, 75]. The results of calculation and their comparison with experimental data are shown in Figs 49-53.

As it can be seen in these figures, there is only one good agreement between calculation and experiment at T = 308 K (Fig. 49). In the other figures (Figs.50-52) the variation of ΔH is different for calculated and experimental values. Thus, in Fig.53 there is a change of enthalpy behavior. This is apparently due to the fact that the solubility data for the system (caffeine – SC-CO_2) can vary.

In Figs.53-54 are shown the measurements and comparisons of the mixing enthalpy of SC-CO_2 in aqueous solution of caffeine.

According to the rule of Sementchenko [93] characteristics of molecular fields of the system's components define the characteristics of the phase equilibrium (Figure 55, 56).

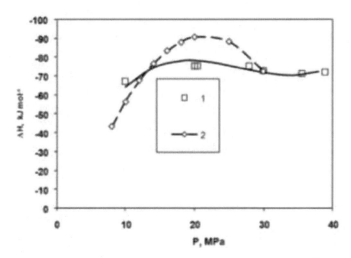

Figure 49. Comparison of the enthalpy of dissolution (ΔH) of caffeine in SC-CO_2 with calculation using the formula (5) at temperature T = 308 K: 1 – experiment; 2 – calculation according to [32].

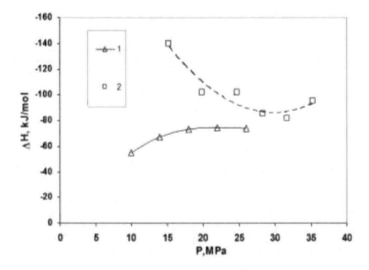

Figure 50. Comparison of the enthalpy of dissolution (ΔH) of caffeine in SC-CO$_2$ with calculation using the formula (5) at temperature T = 323 K: 1 – experiment; 2 – calculation according to [87].

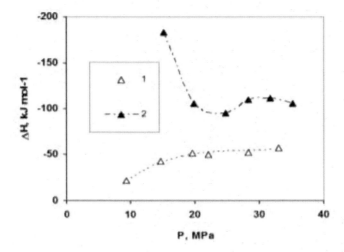

Figure 51. Comparison of the enthalpy of dissolution (ΔH) of caffeine in SC-CO$_2$ with calculation using the formula (5) at temperature T = 323 K: 1 – experiment; 2 – calculation according to [87].

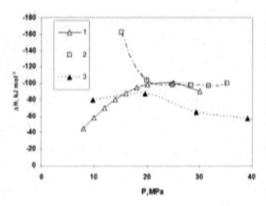

Figure 52. Comparison of the enthalpy of dissolution (ΔH) of caffeine in SC-CO_2 at temperature T = 330 K with calculation using the formula (5) by different authors: 1 – [32]; 2 – [87]; 3 – [51].

CONCLUSION

Three procedures for raw tea pretreatment using supercritical carbon dioxide have been proposed (static, dynamic, decompression), in order to change the structure of a tea leaf and also to use the biological potential more efficiently at the level of beverage concoction. The experimental conditions were determined for the extraction of caffeine, in order to ensure the necessary swelling of a tea leaf with a minimal transport of this important component, by carbon dioxide in dynamic procedure (7.0-10.0 MPa, 305-330 K). For the samples of tea leaves treated as discussed previously, there is a 20-35 % increase in mass transfer of caffeine in aqueous phase at the stage of beverage concoction.

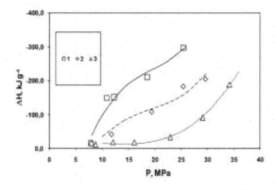

Figure 53. Comparison of the enthalpy of dissolution (ΔH) of caffeine aqueous solution in SC-CO_2 at various temperatures as a function of pressure: 1 – T = 308 K; 2 – T = 323 K; 3 – T = 343 K.

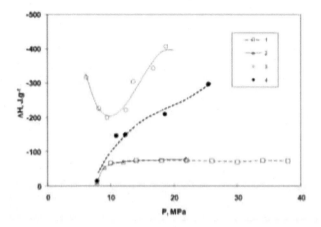

Figure 54. The enthalpies of dissolution (ΔH) of the system SC-CO_2 -: 1 – caffeine (T = 308K); 2 – cellulose (T = 308 K); 3 – tea leaf (T = 304,4 K); 4 – aqueous solution of caffeine (T = 308 K).

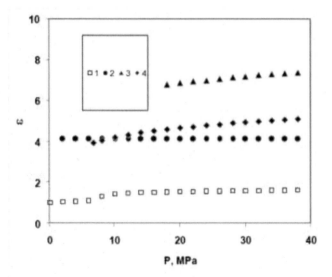

Figure 55. Dielectric capacity of components at T =308 K as a function of pressure: 1 – SC-CO_2 [94]; 2 – caffeine [95]; 3 – aqueous solution of CO_2 (90%) (T = 304,4K); 4 – aqueous solution of CO_2 (94%).

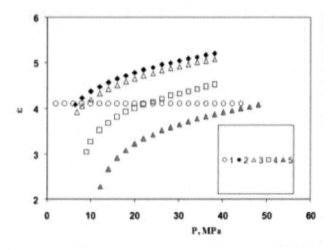

Figure 56. Dielectric capacity of caffeine and aqueous solution of CO_2 as a function of pressure and temperature: 1 – caffeine [95]; 2 – aqueous solution of CO_2 (T = 305 K); 3 – aqueous solution of CO_2 (T = 308K); 4 – aqueous solution of CO_2 (T = 323K); 5 – aqueous solution of CO_2 (T = 343 K).

The swelling of tea leaves and cellulose in SC-CO_2 medium has been analyzed and evaluated using the methods of microscopy and IR-Fourier absorption spectroscopy. The differences in hydrogen bond networks of a tea leaf and one of its components, the cellulose are noticeable. We have also found that there are abundantly stronger hydrogen bonds in tea leaves and that the treatment du CO_2 leads to a decrease in the number of O-H···O groups, which absorb in the area of 3390 cm^{-1}.

The morphology and size characteristics of the fraction of caffeine, dissolved in SC-CO_2 and precipitated from raw tea within the decompression procedures, were modeled by the RESS process, for the system (caffeine - SC-CO_2). With the increase of pressure, the level of dispersion of caffeine increases. A corresponding increase in the phase surface is responsible for the increase in dissolution of caffeine in aqueous solution at the stage of beverage concoction.

It was found that the static treatment of raw tea by SC-CO_2 does not change its elemental composition. Supercritical fluid extraction technology allows obtaining all extracts and ingredients as the traditional technologies, but of higher quality and predictable composition. All supercritical extracts possess more rich composition of natural ingredients comparing to processes produced with the use of organic solvents and do not contain foreign admixtures. The selection of appropriate operating conditions and possibly of some other important target components, can contribute to more efficient use of the natural potential of tea leaves, in manufacturing ingredients for food, pharmaceutical, cosmetics and perfumery industries

ACKNOWLEDGMENTS

The research was performed in a "Joint scientific-educational center for training specialists in the field of critical phenomena and supercritical fluid technologies" SEI HVE "Kazan National Research Technological University", OJSC "Tatneftekhiminvest-Holding", "Supercritical technology" Ltd with a financial support by RFBR (grants number 09-03-12135-ofi-m and 13-3-12078).

The authors are grateful to Fakhreev A.K., Remizov A.B. and Usmanov R.A. for the discussion of results and valuable pieces of advice.

REFERENCES

[1] Chahova E.I., Tatarchenko T.I., Kasianov G. Improving the manufacturing technology of tea. *Izvestia vuzov. pischevaya tehnologia,* 2003, pp.11–15.

[2] Cansell F, Petitet J.P. Fluides Supercritiques et Materiaux, *LIMHP CNRS.* 1995; 372 p.

[3] Zosel K. Process for recovering caffeine, U.S. Patent 3.806.619 (1974).

[4] Zosel K.. Separation with supercritical gases: practical applications. *Angewandte Chemie International Edition* 1978; 17:702–715.

[5] Zosel K. Separation with supercritical gases: practical applications, in: Schneider G, Stahl E, Wilke G. (Eds.). *Extraction with Supercritical Gases,* Weinheim,Verlag Chemie 1980, p. 123.

[6] Zosel K. Process for the decaffeination of coffee, U.S. Patent 4.247.570 (1981).

[7] Zosel K. Process for the direct decaffeination of aqueous coffee extract solutions. U.S. Pa-tent 4.348.422 (1982).

[8] Roseluis W, Vitzthum O, Hubert P. Method for the production of caffeine-free coffee ex-tract. U.S. Patent 3.843.824 (1974).

[9] Vitzthum O, Hubert P. Process for the decaffeination of raw coffee. U.S. Patent 3.879.569 (1975).

[10] Prasad R, Gottesman M, Scarella R.A., Decaffeination of aqueous extracts. U.S. Patent 4.246.291 (1981).

[11] Margolis G, Chiovini J. Decaffeination process, U.S. Patent 4.251.559 (1981).

[12] Roselius L., Kurzhals H.A. Method for the selective extraction of caffeine from vegetable materials. U.S. Patent 4.255.458 (1981).

[13] Jasovsky G.A., Gottesman M. Preparation of a decaffeinated roasted coffee blend. U.S. Pa-tent 4.255.461 (1981).

[14] Peter S, Brunner G. Process for decaffeinating coffee. U.S. Patent 4.322.445 (1982).

[15] Prasad R., Gottesman M., Scarella R.A. Decaffeination of aqueous roasted coffee extract. U.S. Patent 4.341.804 (1982).

[16] Hubert P., Vitzthum O. Process for the extraction of caffeine from super-critical solutions. U.S. Patent 4.411.923 (1983).

[17] Katz S.N. Decaffeination process. U.S. Patent 4.472.442 (1984).

[18] Katz S.N. Method for decaffeinating coffee with a supercritical fluid. U.S. Patent 4.820.537 (1989).

[19] Hermsen M., Sirtl W. Process for decaffeination of raw coffee. U.S. Patent 5.135.766 (1992).

[20] Vitzthum O, Hubert P. Method for the manufacture of caffeine free black tea. U.S. Patent 4.167.589 (1979).

[21] Gebrig M., Forster A. Process for the production of decaffeinated tea. U.S. Patent 4.938.977 (1990).

[22] Klima H., Schitz E., Vollbrecht H.R. Process for the decaffeination of tea. U.S. Patent 4.976.979 (1990).

[23] Schulmeyr J. Process for aromatization of treated tea. U.S. Patent 5.087.468 (1992).

[24] Park H.S., Lee H.J., Shin M.H., Lee K.W., Lee H., Kim Y.S., Kim K.O., Kim K.H. The effects of co-solvents on the decaffeination of green tea by supercritical carbon dioxide. *Food Chemistry* 2007; 105: 1011–1017.

[25] Armstrong R.G., Deszyck E.J., Madures J.W., Young R.H. Process for puffing tobacco. U.S. Patent 3.771.533 (1973).

[26] Lowry G.R. Tobacco expansion process and apparatus. U.S. Patent 4.870.980 (1989).

[27] Saputra D., Pane F.A., Cornelius P.L. Puffing dehydrated green bell peppers with carbon dioxide. *American Society of Agricultural Engineers* 1991; 34: 475–480.

Utilization Efficiency Improvement ... 197

[28] Stahl E., Rau G., Carius W. Cracking and puffing of plant material by CO_2 high pressure treatment. *Zeitschrift for lebensmittel-untersuchung und-forschung* 1986; 182: 33–35.

[29] Gumerov F.M., Sabirzianov A.N., Gumerova G.I. *Sub- and Supercritical Fluids in Polymers Processing*, 2000, Kazan, 328 p.

[30] Truong N.H., Fakhreev A.K., Gumerov F.M., Gabitov F.R., Usmanov R.A., Amirkhanov D.G., Yarullin R.S. The implementation of supercritical carbon dioxide in order to improve consumer properties and the economic factors of Vietnamese green tea production, *Supercritical Fluids. Theory and practice* 2008; 3; 2: 7-19.

[31] Shamsetdinov F.N., Yarullin L.Yu., Gumerov F.M., Gabitov F.R., Zaripov Z.I, Remizov A.B., Kolyadko I.M., Nikitin V.G., Fakhreev A.K., Kamalova D.I. Effect of treatment in supercritical CO_2 on the composition and structure of tea leaf and cellulose. *Russian Journal of Physical Chemistry* 2011; 5; 7: 1167-1172.

[32] Truong N.H. Gumerov F., Gabitov F., Usmanov R., Hairutdinov V., Le Neindre B. Improvement of the water brewing of Vietnamese green tea by pretreatment with supercritical carbon dioxide. *J. of Supercritical Fluids* 2012; 62: 73-78.

[33] Burgos-Solyrzano G.I., Brennecke J.F., Stadtherr M.A. Solubility measurements and mode-ling of molecules of biological and pharmaceutical interest with supercritical CO_2. *Fluid Phase Equilibrium* 2004; 220: 55–67.

[34] Mary Den Idz. Vitamins and Mineral Substances, *Eds. "Complect"*, St. Petersburg, 1995 (in Russian).

[35] Ksibi H., Moussa A.B., Baccar M. Powder structure transition under the recrystallization conditions in the RESS process. *Chem.Eng.Technol.* 2006; 29; 7: 868-874.

[36] Gilmutdinov I.M., Sabirzyanov A.N., Gumerov F.M. The effect of solvent's density and channel's geometry on the morphology and size of the obtained micro-particles in the process of rapid expansion of the supercritical solution. *Supercritical Fluids. Theory and practice* 2008; 3; 1: 43-49.

[37] Gilmutdinov I.M., Khairutdinov V.F., Kuznetsova I.V., Mukhamadiev A.A., Gabitov F.R., Gumerov F.M., Sabirzyanov A.N. The Dispersion of Polymeric Materials with the Use of Supercritical Fluids. *Russian Journal of Physical Chemistry B* 2009; 3; 8: 1145–1153.

[38] Zelepugin D.Yu., Til'kunova N.A., Chernishova I.V. The use of supercritical fluids for nano-and microforms of pharmaceutical substances. *Supercritical fluids. Theory and practice* 2008; 3; 1: 5-23.

[39] Zhbankov R.G. Infrared Spectra of Cellulose and its Derivatives, «Nauka Tekhnika», Minsk, 1964 (in Russian).

[40] GOST 30178-96. «Raw Materials and Food Stuffs. Atomic Absorption Method for the De-termination of Toxic Elements».

[41] GOST 30692-2000. *«Feed, Feed Milling Raw Materials. Atomic Absorption Method for the Determination of Content of Copper, Lead, Zinc, and Cadmium».*

[42] GOST 26929-94. *"Raw Materials and Food-Stuffs. Preparation of Samples. Mineralization for the Determination of Toxic Element Content".*

[43] Iogansen A.V., *Spectrochim. Acta. Part A* 1999; 55: p. 1582.

[44] GOST R 52930-2008. "Vodka, special vodka and water for the concoction. Mass concentration definition of cations, amines, inorganic anions and organic acids by capillary electrophoresis method".

[45] Ziaedini A,. Jafari A., Zakeri A. Extraction of antioxidants and caffeine from green tea (Camelia sinensis) leaves: Kinetics and modeling. *Food Science and Technology International* 2010; 16: 505-510.

[46] Kwang J.L., Sang H.L. Extraction Behavior of Caffeine and EGCG from Green and Black Tea. *Biotechnology and Bioprocess Engineering* 2008; 13: 646-649.

[47] Xi Jun, Shen Deji, Li Ye, Zhang Rui. Comparison of in vitro antioxidant activities and bio-active components of green tea extracts by different extraction methods. *International Journal of Pharmaceutics* 2011; 408: 97–101.

[48] Koschel D., Coxam J.Y. Enthalpy and solubility data of CO_2 in water and NaCl (aq.) at conditions of interest for geological sequestration. *Fluid Phase Equilibrium* 2006; 247: p.107.

[49] Koschel D., Coxam J.Y., Majer V. *Ind. Eng. Chem. Res.,* 2007; 46: p. 1421.

[50] Mathonat C., Majer V., Mather A.E., Grolier J.P. *Fluid Phase Equilibrium* 1997; 40: p.171.

[51] Kim J.R., Kyong J.B., *Bul.Korean Chem.Soc.,* 1995; 16; 5: p.432.

[52] Grolier J.P., Wilhelm E. *Pure &Appl. Chem.,* 1991; 63; 10: 1427-1434.

[53] *Walas S.M. Phase Equilibria in Chemical Engineering.* Butterworth-Heinemann. Boston. 1985.

[54] Sanchez C., Lacombe R.H. An Elementary Molecular Theory of Classical Fluids. Pure Fluids. *The Journal of Physical Chemistry,* 1976; 80; 21: 2352-2362.

[55] Sanchez C, Lacombe R.H. Thermodynamics of Polymer Solutions. *Macromolecules* 1978; 11; 6: 1145-1155.

[56] Vrentad J.S., Vrentas C.M. Sorption in Glassy Polymers. *Macromolecules,* 1991; 24: 2404-2412.

[57] Calvet E., Prat A. *Microcalorimetry. Implementation in physical chemistry and biology.* Foreign. lit. Moscow 1963.

[58] Zaripov Z.I., Burtsev S.A., Gavrilov A.V, Mukhamedzyanov GKh. Thermal Properties of n-Hexane at Temperatures of 298.15–363.5 K and Pressures of 0.098–147 MPa. *Theoretical Foundations of Chemical Engineering,* 2002; 36; 4: 400–405.

[59] Zaripov Z.I., Burtsev S.A., Gavrilov A.V., Mukhamedzyanov GKh. Determination of the Thermophysical Properties of Halogenated Hydrocarbons in a Heat-Conducting Calorimeter. *High Temperature,* 2004; 42; 2: 282–289.

[60] Zaripov Z.I., Burtsev S.A., Bulaev S.A., Mukhamedzyanov G.Kh. The Heat Capacity and Thermal Diffusivity of Aqueous Solutions of Alkali Metal Salts in a Wide Pressure Range *J. Phys. Chem.,* 2004; 78; 5: 697-700.

[61] Zaripov Z.I., Mukhamedzyanov G.Kh. Thermophysical properties of liquids and solutions: (monograph). Kazan state technological university. Kazan. 2008.

[62] Liu L., Peng Q, Y. Li. *Inorganic Chem.,* 2008; 47: 5022-5028.

[63] Ayele D.W., Chen H.M., Su W.N., Pan C.J., Chen L.Y., Chou H.L., Cheng J.H., Hwang B.J., Lee J.F. *Chem. Eur. J.,* 2011; 17: 5737–5744.

[64] D.W. van Krevelen, Nijenhuis K. Properties of Polymers Structure-Property Correlations of Polymers Estimation and Prediction of Properties of Polymers Functional Structural Groups in Polymers Additive Group. *Contributions in Polymers.* Elsevier, 2009, 1004p.

[65] Bayer E, Hiltner A. *High-molecular compounds* 1996; A series; 38: p. 549.

[66] Kovalenko V.I. Crystalline cellulose: structure and hydrogen bonds. *Chemical success,* 2010; 79; 3: 261-272.

[67] Usmanov R.A., Shamsetdinov F.N., Gabitov R.R. and others. The effect of SC-CO_2 treatment procedures on content and structure of a tea leaf and cellulose. *Supercritical fluids: theory and practice,* 2011; 6; 2: 83–91.

[68] Uriyash V.F., Larina V.N., Kokurina N.Y., Novoselova N.V. Thermochemical characteristics of cellulose and its aqueous mixtures. *Journal of physical chemistry,* 2010; 84; 6: 1023-1029.

[69] Eoyelovich M.Ya. Enthalpy of formation and dissolution of cellulose. Union Conference on Chemical Thermodynamics and calorimetry (thesis). *Gorkiy GGU* 1988; Part 2: 189-191.

[70] NIST.gov: National institute of standards and technology (Electronic source). USA. Thermophysical properties of liquids 2011.

[71] Dordain L., Coxam J.Y., Grolier J.P. Measurement of isobaric heat capacities of gases from 323.15 to 573.15 K up to 30 MPa. *Rev. Sci. Instrum.,* 1994; 65; 10: 3263-3267.

[72] Cesaro A., Staree G. Thermodynamic Properties of Caffeine Cristal. *J. Phys. Chem.,* 1980; 84: 1345-1346.

[73] Bothe H., Cammenga H.G. Phase transitions and thermodynamic properties of anhydrous caffeine. *Journal of Thermal Analysis,* 1979; 16: 267-275.

[74] Attllio C.B, Giorglo Starec. Thermodynamic Properties of Caffeine Crystal Forms. *J. Phys. Chem.,* 1980; 84: 1345-1346.

[75] Griesser U.J., Szelagiewicz M., Hofmeier U.Ch., Pitt C., Cianferani S. Vapor pressure and heat of sublimation of crystal polymorphs. *Journal of Thermal Analysis and Calorimetry,* 1999; 57: 45-60.

[76] Defossemont G., Stanislaw L., Randzio S.L., Legendre B. Contributions of Calorimetry for *Cp* Determination and of Scanning Transitiometry for the Study of Polymorphism. *Crystal Growth & Design,* 2004; 4 (6): 1169-1174.

[77] Emel'yanenko V.N., Verevkin S.P. Thermodynamic properties of caffeine: Reconciliation of available experimental data. *J. Chem. Thermodynamics,* 2008; 40: 1661–1665.

[78] Dong J.X., Li Q., Tan Z.C., Zhang Z.H., Liu Y. The standard molar enthalpy of formation, molar heat capacities, and thermal stability of anhydrous caffeine. *J. Chem. Thermodynamics,* 2007; 39: 108–114.

[79] Fen XU, Shu QIU, Jun LIANG Jian, Guo WU Rui, Hua SUN Li, Xian LI Fen. Low temperature heat capacity and thermal analysis of caffeine. Theophylline and Aminophylline. *Acta Phys. Chem. Sin.,* 2010; 26(8): 2096-2102.

[80] Shamsetdinov F.N., Bulaev S.A., Zaripov Z.I. Thermophysical properties of supercritical carbon dioxide – caffeine system. *Herald of Kazan state technological university,* 2010; 11: 465-468.

[81] Deiters U.K., Randzio S.L. A combined determination of phase diagrams of asymmetric binary mixtures by equations of state and transitiometry. *Fluid Phase Equilibrium,* 2007; 260: 87–97.

[82] Stern J.H., Lowe E.. Enthalpies of Transfer of Theophylline and Caffeine from Water to Aqueous Alcohols at 25 C. *Journal of Chemical and Engineering Data,* 1978; 23; 4: 341-342.

[83] Stern J.H., Beeninga L.R. Partial Molar Heat Capacities of Caffeine and Theophylline in Pure water. *The Journal of Physical Chemistry,* 1975; 79; 6: 582-584.

[84] Stokkeland I., Skauge L.A., Htiland H. Changes in Partial Molar Volume and Isentropic Partial Molar Compressibility of Self-Association of Purine and Caffeine in Aqueous Solution at 1-1600 Bar. *Journal of Solution Chemistry,* 1986; 16: 1.

[85] Su C.S., Chen Y.P. Correlation for the solubility of pharmaceutical compounds in supercritical carbon dioxide. *Fluid Phase Equilibrium,* 2007; 254: 167–173.

[86] Johannsen M., Brunner G. Solubility of the xanthines caffeine, theophylline and theobromine in supercritical carbon dioxide. *Fluid Phase Equilibrium,* 1994; 95: 215-26.

[87] Azevedo Á.B.A. et al. Supercritical CO_2 recovery of caffeine from green coffee oil: new experimental solubility data and modeling. *Quím. Nova [online]* 2008; 31; 6: 1319-1323.

[88] Usmanov R.A., Gumerov F.M., Gabitov F.R., Zaripov Z.I, Shamsetdinov F.N., Abdulagatov I.M. High Yield Biofuel Production from Vegetable Oils with Supercritical Alcohols (monograph). *Liquid fuels: Types, properties and production* (section 3): Nova Science Publishers. NY. 2012.

[89] Usmanov R.A., Shamsetdinov F.N., Gabitov R.R., Biktashev Sh.A., Gumerov F.M., Gabitov F.R., Zaripov Z.I., Gazizov R.A., Yarullin L.Y., Yakushev I.A. Pilot plant for the continuous transesterification of vegetable oils in supercritical methanol, ethanol. *Supercritical fluids: theory and practice* 2011; 2: 1–19.

[90] Vasilyev I.A., Petrov V.M. Thermodynamic properties of oxigen-containing organic compounds. *Chemistry.* Leningrad. 1984. 240 p.

[91] Naziyev Ya.M., Shahverdiev A.N., Bashirov M.M., Aliyev N.S. Thermo-properties of single-atom esters (isobaric heat capacity). *TVT* 1994; 32; 6: p.936.

[92] Zaripov Z.I., Burtsev S.A., Gavrilov A.V., Bulaev S.A., Mukhamedzyanov G.Kh. Thermal and calorimetric properties of n-butyl ester. *Herald of Kazan technological university,* 2002; 1-2: 208-212.

[93] Karapetyan M.H. Introduction to the theory of chemical processes. Moscow. *Higher school.* 1975. p. 320.

[94] NIST. REFPROP Standard Reference Database 23, Version 9.0 REFPROP

INDEX

A

absorption spectra, 155
absorption spectroscopy, 194
abuse, ix, 64, 65, 89, 90, 91, 92, 98, 107, 108
access, 22, 25, 41, 93, 94, 96, 107
accessibility, 152, 167
acetaldehyde, 103
acetaminophen, 73, 86
acid, 10, 43, 47, 50, 54, 77, 115, 118, 119, 122, 127, 167, 182, 183
acidosis, 57, 58
activated carbon, 142
acupuncture, 77
acute migraine, ix, 36
AD, 82
adaptation, 60, 72, 138
ADC, 178
adenosine, ix, 6, 7, 13, 15, 30, 33, 39, 40, 41, 47, 48, 49, 50, 60, 63, 64, 66, 71, 72, 77, 81, 85, 90, 94, 95, 103, 104, 105, 106, 108, 109, 110, 132, 134, 136
ADHD, 31
adiponectin, 115, 129
adipose, 115, 130
adipose tissue, 115, 130
adjustment, 59
adolescents, 53, 54
adrenaline, 129

adulthood, 97
adults, viii, 12, 16, 20, 35, 54, 56, 65, 68, 92, 128
adverse effects, 37, 48, 49, 51, 53, 56, 63, 77
Africa, 41
African-American, 53
age, ix, 2, 3, 4, 9, 13, 14, 16, 17, 35, 37, 39, 56, 58, 71, 72, 73, 93, 97
albumin, 38
alcohol abuse, 110
alcohol addiction, ix, 90
alcohol consumption, ix, 34, 51, 70, 90, 92, 93, 98, 101, 103, 111
alcohol dependence, 70, 79, 93, 103
alcohol withdrawal, ix, 90
alcoholism, 91, 104, 105
alertness, ix, 6, 10, 15, 18, 35, 47, 48, 60, 63, 64, 69, 71, 72, 85, 99, 110
alkaloids, 42
alkalosis, 49
alters, 4, 140
American Psychiatric Association, 67, 69, 83, 93, 103
amines, 166, 197
amino, 63, 175
amino acid(s), 63, 175
ammonia, 62, 141
amygdala, 31
amyloid beta, 13
analgesic, 48, 71, 73, 74, 77, 86

Index

anaphylaxis, 53
anorexia, 57
ANOVA, 25, 26, 27, 96
antagonism, 13, 30, 39, 41, 47, 49, 64, 94, 103, 107, 109, 132
antibody, 119
anticholinergic, 16
antidepressants, 76
antioxidant, 6, 13, 75, 153, 198
anxiety, 53, 54, 56, 60, 63, 65, 66, 69, 70, 83, 91, 95, 96, 97, 99, 105, 107, 109, 110, 111
anxiety disorder, 65
apnea, ix, 35, 49, 71, 80, 85
apoptosis, 5, 6, 132
appetite, 20, 33
aqueous solutions, 175, 181
arousal, 12, 28, 56, 72, 90
arrhythmia, 49
arsenic, 153
arterial blood gas, 57
Asia, 140
assessment, 11, 74, 78
assimilation, 153
asthma, 79, 80
athletes, 2, 4, 5, 10, 62, 63, 72
atmospheric pressure, 182
atopy, 54
ATP, 121
atrial fibrillation, 48, 53, 81
atrial flutter, 53
avoidance, 6

B

bacteria, 152
barbiturates, 57, 58, 77
barium, 167
basal metabolic rate, 40
base, 29
basic research, 50
BD, 83
behavioral effects, ix, 28, 60, 90, 107
bending, 158, 159
beneficial effect, 59, 101, 115

benefits, 6, 59, 85
benzodiazepine, 40
beverages, vii, 2, 9, 10, 11, 36, 37, 41, 49, 53, 60, 79, 83, 85, 90, 93, 102, 104, 107, 109, 110, 115, 132, 140
bile, 39, 50
biliary tract, 50
binge drinking, 93, 98, 102
bioavailability, 38, 77
biological activity, 39
biopolymer, 143, 179
bipolar disorder, 66
black tea, 140, 141, 142, 174, 196
blood, 2, 7, 14, 15, 17, 18, 37, 38, 48, 49, 55, 56, 57, 62, 80, 93, 95, 98, 101, 115, 120, 124, 129, 136
blood flow, 48, 49
blood pressure, 2, 17, 18, 48, 49, 56, 62, 80, 136
blood-brain barrier, 7, 14, 15
body mass index, 76
body size, 56, 72, 73
body weight, 10, 20, 51, 56
bonding, 158
bonds, 158, 160
bone, 50, 54
bowel, 57
bowel sounds, 57
brain, 6, 7, 8, 14, 15, 32, 38, 47, 64, 83, 105, 106, 115
branching, 14
breakdown, 10
breast milk, 39, 52
breastfeeding, 52
breathing, 50, 54
bronchodilator, 49
bronchopulmonary dysplasia, 71
brothers, 56
burn, 62

C

Ca^{2+}, x, 114, 118, 119, 121, 125, 126, 134, 135, 167
cacao, vii, 36, 37, 42, 44

Index

cadmium, 154

caffeine use, vii, 1, 2, 3, 8, 11, 16, 20, 54, 59, 60, 61, 67, 69, 70, 73, 74, 80, 107, 128, 181

caffeine-ethanol interactions, ix, 89

calcium, 2, 4, 7, 40, 50, 58, 134, 153, 167

caloric intake, 20

calorimetric measurements, 175

calorimetry, 199

campaigns, 90, 102

cancer, 55, 59, 74, 86, 133, 140

cancer death, 59

capillary, 166, 197

carbamazepine, 76, 77

carbohydrate(s), 4, 6, 11, 12, 14, 18, 62, 63, 85

carbon, xi, 49, 71, 139, 141, 142, 144, 146, 147, 148, 149, 151, 152, 153, 154, 160, 162, 166, 169, 170, 174, 175, 176, 179, 181, 191, 196, 200

carbon dioxide, xi, 49, 71, 139, 141, 142, 144, 146, 147, 148, 149, 151, 152, 153, 154, 160, 162, 166, 169, 170, 174, 175, 176, 179, 181, 191, 196, 200

cardiac arrhythmia, 53, 66, 67, 80

cardiovascular disease, 59, 140

cardiovascular system, 71

catecholamines, 40, 41, 47, 51, 111

causality, 17, 54

causation, 122, 127

C-C, 175

cell cycle, 55

cell membranes, 37, 38

cell surface, 39

cellular energy, x, 114, 121

cellulose, xi, 140, 143, 152, 154, 155, 158, 159, 160, 166, 175, 179, 180, 181, 192, 194, 196, 199

central nervous system, 32, 39, 47, 62, 71, 94

cerebellum, 64

cerebral blood flow, 48

cerebral cortex, 64

cerebrospinal fluid, 7

certificate, 154, 166, 176

chemical, viii, xi, 35, 43, 139, 143, 146, 201

children, 37, 54, 56

China, vii, 36, 128

chlorine, 153

chocolate, vii, 36, 37, 44, 63

cholesterol, 7, 14, 50, 76

choroid, 7

chromatography, 31, 170

chronic diseases, 115

cigarette smoke, 91

cigarette smokers, 91

cigarette smoking, 85, 91, 104

cimetidine, 76

circulation, xi, 139, 144, 154, 155, 159, 161, 166, 172, 173

cirrhosis, 74, 86

City, 17

classes, 29

classification, 68, 106

clinical symptoms, 66

clozapine, 76, 77

CNS, 47, 56, 63, 64, 66, 68, 71, 72, 84

coaches, 73

cobalt, 155, 156, 157

cocaine, 21, 29, 31, 32, 33, 34, 68, 91, 105, 106, 110

cocoa, 63

Coffea arabica, vii, 36, 41

Coffea canephora, vii, 36

cognition, vii, 1, 6, 7, 8, 9, 16, 18, 34

cognitive abilities, 64

cognitive deficit9s), 6, 13

cognitive function, 6, 13, 15, 16, 17, 60, 72

cognitive impairment, vii, 1, 8, 14, 16

cognitive performance, 17, 18, 74, 110

cognitive process, 8

cognitive processing, 8

coke, 54, 82

college campuses, 90

college students, 90, 92, 103, 104, 107, 108

colorectal cancer, 55

coma, 57, 58

combined effect, 18

commercial, xi, 37, 43, 139, 143

common symptoms, 69

community, 17, 54, 104
comparative analysis, 146
competition, 62
complications, 37, 53
composition, xi, 140, 146, 152, 153, 154, 155, 166, 194, 196
compounds, 158, 177, 181, 199, 200
compression, 177
computer, 22, 178
conditioned stimulus, 23
conditioning, 23, 24, 144, 166, 167, 169, 170, 172
confounders, viii, 2, 59
congestive heart failure, 50, 75
congress, 107
connectivity, 7, 15
consensus, 100
conservation, 175
consolidation, 15
consumers, 4, 9, 15, 31, 49, 63, 68, 69, 70, 90, 93, 98, 99, 100, 102, 104, 120
consumption patterns, 108
contraceptives, 76
control group, 96
controlled studies, 69, 70
controversial, 20
cooling, 155
coordination, 99, 100, 108
copper, 153, 154, 156, 157
coronary heart disease, 54
correlation(s), 91, 189
corticotropin, 34
cosmetics, 140, 194
cost, 71, 141, 144
craving, 69
creatine, 63, 121
crystalline, 160
crystals, 167
CSF, 7
cues, 21, 26, 28, 29, 30, 33
cycles, 97
cycling, 2, 4, 10, 12, 18
CYP inhibitors, viii, 35
cytochrome, viii, 35, 39, 56, 74, 76
cytokines, 115

D

danger, 63
data collection, 22
deaths, 55
decontamination, 57, 58
deficiency, 6, 153
deficit, 31, 64
deformation, 158
degradation, 85
dehydration, 101
dementia, vii, 1, 6, 7, 8, 9, 13, 16
dendrites, 14
Denmark, 2, 102
dependent variable, 96
deposition, 160
depression, vii, ix, 1, 9, 17, 35, 65, 69, 95, 99, 111
depressive symptoms, 17, 54
deprivation, x, 93, 104, 114, 123, 124
derivatives, 40
detectable, 52, 95, 122
detection, 31, 60
deviation, 177, 181, 182, 184
diabetes, 52, 115, 128, 130, 136
Diagnostic and Statistical Manual of Mental Disorders, 67, 69, 83, 93, 103
diagnostic criteria, 65, 67, 68
diaphoresis, 66
diarrhea, 57
diastolic blood pressure, 53
diet, vii, ix, 6, 7, 8, 14, 35, 36, 37, 39, 40, 45, 54, 63, 82, 87, 93, 129, 132, 136
diffusion, 116, 175
diffusivity, 141
direct action, 94
direct measure, 28, 175
discrimination, 6, 13, 29, 84
discrimination training, 29
discriminative stimuli, 29, 33
diseases, 14, 115, 153, 167
disinfection, 167
disorder, 31, 48, 60, 65, 66, 68, 84
dispersion, 154, 194
distilled water, 146, 174

Index

distress, 67, 69
distribution, viii, 35, 38, 127
diuretic, ix, 35, 49, 50, 62, 75
dizziness, 69, 70, 100
DNA, 55
DNA repair, 55
dogs, 80
DOI, 80, 85
dopamine, 30, 31, 32, 33, 34, 47, 104
dopaminergic, 6, 30, 31, 60, 64, 66, 104
dose-response relationship, 51
drinking water, 91, 97
drug dependence, 85, 95, 108
drug interaction, 56
drug metabolism, 56
drugs, ix, 37, 55, 56, 76, 77, 83, 90, 91, 92, 100, 109
drying, 141, 143, 146
DSM-IV-TR, 65, 66, 68, 69
dual task, 60
duodenal ulcer, 54
dyspepsia, 50

E

edema, 50, 75
editors, 84
electroconvulsive therapy, ix, 36
electrolyte, 63
electron, 121, 144
electrophoresis, 166, 197
emergency, 60, 74
endocrine, ix, 35
endurance, 2, 3, 4, 11, 12, 17, 61, 62, 90, 136
energy, ix, x, 11, 18, 20, 31, 34, 37, 40, 44, 53, 55, 56, 59, 75, 79, 89, 90, 92, 93, 95, 98, 99, 100, 101, 102, 103, 104, 105, 106, 108, 109, 110, 111, 114, 118, 121, 123, 124, 127, 138, 144, 159
energy drinks, ix, 11, 31, 37, 44, 55, 56, 79, 89, 90, 92, 93, 95, 98, 99, 100, 101, 102, 104, 108, 109, 111
energy expenditure, 138
England, 9

environment, 21, 153
environmental factors, 38
environmental stimuli, viii, 20, 28
enzymes, 6, 39, 40, 48
epidemiologic, 9, 10, 51
epidemiologic studies, 10, 51
epigenetics, 15
equality, 189
equilibrium, 145, 146, 154, 175, 190
equipment, xi, 140, 166, 176
ester, 201
ethanol, ix, 29, 89, 92, 93, 94, 95, 97, 99, 101, 103, 104, 105, 106, 107, 108, 109, 201
ethanol metabolism, 94
ethyl acetate, 141
etiology, 72, 104
European Commission, 101, 105
evidence, ix, x, 9, 17, 30, 35, 49, 50, 53, 54, 65, 68, 74, 84, 104, 114
exaggeration, 56, 66
excitation, 47, 58, 125
excretion, 2
exercise, vii, 1, 2, 3, 4, 5, 6, 8, 11, 12, 13, 17, 61, 62, 63, 72, 115, 116, 117, 127, 129, 130, 131, 135, 136, 137, 138
exercise performance, vii, 1, 11, 12, 61, 72
exercise-related pain, vii, 1
exertion, 5, 12, 13
experimental condition, 191
exposure, viii, 20, 21, 28, 30, 34, 50, 51, 52, 55, 65, 71, 95, 101, 104, 106, 110, 132, 151
extinction, 20, 21, 23, 24, 25, 26, 27, 28, 29, 30, 33, 34
extinction phase, 24, 25
extraction, xi, 139, 141, 142, 144, 148, 149, 152, 175, 192, 195, 198
extracts, 194, 195, 198

F

fat, 6, 23, 26, 28, 30, 45, 62, 129, 130, 136
fatty acids, 10, 40, 131
FDA, 37, 55, 101

fear, 53, 64
federal law, 102
feedstock, xi, 139, 144, 171
feelings, 60, 99, 100
fertility, 51
fetal growth, 52
fever, 57
fiber, 127, 138
fibrillation, 53
fights, 60
filtration, 49
financial, 194
financial support, 194
fitness, 110
fixed-interval schedule, 33
flavor, 141
flaws, 51
flex, 3
flowers, 43
fluid, 50, 63, 81, 142, 143, 144, 146, 153, 154, 175, 178, 194, 195
fluid balance, 81
fluid extract, 146, 154, 194
fluoxetine, 76
fluvoxamine, 76, 77
food, viii, 19, 20, 21, 22, 23, 24, 25, 26, 27, 28, 29, 30, 31, 32, 33, 34, 41, 42, 52, 91, 94, 102, 105, 142, 153, 154, 167, 194
food additive, 102
Food and Drug Administration, 37, 101, 102
food intake, 20, 34, 94, 105
food-seeking behavior, viii, 20, 21, 27, 29, 30, 32, 33
food-seeking responses, viii, 20, 21, 24, 26, 29
force, 3, 5, 12
formation, 6, 48, 60, 159, 160, 167, 199, 200
formula, 23, 38, 177, 182, 186, 189, 190, 191
fragments, 6
France, 9, 102, 139
free choice, 94, 107
free volume, 175
fruits, 143

FTIR, 154, 155, 158, 159, 161
funds, 30

G

gallbladder, 50
gallstones, 76
gastroesophageal reflux, 50, 54
gastrointestinal tract, viii, 35, 38
gel, 146
gene expression, 137
genes, 5, 115
genetic factors, ix, 35, 56
genotype, 80
genus, 41
geometry, 197
Germany, 108, 142
gestational diabetes, 52
ginger, 45
glassy polymers, 175
glomerulus, 49
glucocorticoid, 54
glucocorticoid receptor, 54
glucose, ix, x, 5, 11, 18, 75, 90, 93, 106, 113, 114, 115, 116, 117, 118, 119, 120, 121, 122, 123, 124, 125, 126, 128, 129, 130, 132, 133, 134, 135, 136, 137
glucose tolerance, 75, 127, 129
glucose tolerance test, 129
glucose transport, ix, x, 114, 115, 116, 117, 118, 119, 120, 121, 122, 123, 124, 125, 126, 130, 133, 134, 135, 136
GLUT, 136
GLUT4, 116, 121, 127, 130, 133, 137, 138
glutamate, 103
glycerol, 40
glycine, 34
glycogen, 62, 122, 124, 127, 130, 137
glycolysis, 62
grants, 194
granules, 46
growth, 128
growth factor, 128
guaranine, vii, 36
guidelines, 66

Index

H

half-life, viii, 35, 38, 39, 55, 56, 74
hallucinations, 67
halogen, 144
harmful effects, 68
HE, 82
headache, ix, 35, 47, 54, 69, 70, 73, 74, 82, 86, 100
health, viii, ix, 17, 35, 54, 58, 65, 115, 126, 153, 167
health effects, viii, 35, 58
health problems, 115, 167
health promotion, 126
heart failure, 48, 57, 75, 86
heart rate, 48, 50, 56, 57
heat capacity, xi, 140, 181, 182, 184, 186, 200, 201
hemodialysis, 57, 82
hepatitis, 53
hepatitis a, 53
heroin, 29, 31, 33, 91
heterogeneity, 51
high blood pressure, 52
high fat, viii, 14, 19, 23, 25, 26, 28, 30
hippocampus, 13, 14, 64
history, 48, 55, 57
HM, 12
homeostasis, 40, 116, 118, 128
homocysteine, 51
hormone(s), 51
hormone levels, 51
House, 42
human, vii, ix, 5, 7, 29, 36, 37, 50, 71, 84, 90, 103, 117, 130, 131, 153
human body, vii, 153
human cognition, 7
human subjects, 130
humidity, 21
Hunter, 86
hydrogen, 158, 159, 160, 179, 194, 199
hydrogen bonds, 158, 159, 160, 179, 194, 199
hydroxyl, 158
hydroxyl groups, 158

hyperactivity, 31, 64
hyperemesis, 50
hyperglycaemia, 136
hyperglycemia, 57, 129
hypersomnia, 55, 66
hypertension, 54, 55
hypokalemia, 57
hyponatremia, 82
hypotension, 57, 58
hypothermia, 108
hypothesis, 10, 64, 104, 107
hypoxia, 121, 135, 136

I

ideal, 74, 142
idiopathic, ix, 35
idiosyncratic, 53, 55
illicit drug use, 103
illumination, 23, 24
imbibition, 144, 148, 151, 152
immersion, 154
immunoreactivity, 109
imports, 140
improvements, 61, 72
impulsive, 101
impurities, 158
in vitro, 6, 50, 104, 121, 123, 198
in vivo, 5, 123
incidence, vii, 1, 9, 55, 74, 75, 85, 92, 110, 128
income, 141
incubation period, 119
individuals, vii, 1, 2, 3, 7, 8, 9, 10, 11, 16, 39, 48, 49, 53, 54, 60, 65, 66, 68, 69, 70, 100, 102
indomethacyn, ix, 36
induction, ix, 35, 49, 83
industrial processing, 140
industries, 194
industry, 143
infants, 52
infarction, 57
infertility, 51
inflammation, 59, 75

information processing, 99, 108
ingestion, 2, 3, 4, 6, 7, 8, 9, 10, 11, 12, 13, 17, 18, 37, 49, 55, 56, 57, 63, 81, 106, 109, 117, 120, 127, 129, 130
ingredients, 37, 56, 106, 140, 143, 144, 146, 148, 152, 153, 194
inhibition, x, 7, 39, 41, 47, 48, 71, 76, 114, 121, 127
inhibitor, x, 40, 114, 121, 126, 132
injections, 34, 91, 105, 110
injuries, 80
insecticide, 167
insomnia, 53, 55, 63, 66, 67
insulin, ix, x, 51, 75, 114, 115, 116, 117, 118, 119, 120, 121, 122, 123, 124, 125, 126, 128, 129, 130, 131, 132, 133, 134, 136
insulin resistance, 51, 115, 116, 117, 118, 119, 120, 130, 131, 132, 136
insulin sensitivity, 75, 117, 127, 128, 129, 130, 131, 136
insulin signaling, 115, 117, 118, 119, 120, 130, 131, 133
intoxicating effects, ix, 89, 92, 101
intoxication, 56, 58, 65, 67, 76, 95, 98, 99, 100, 101, 102, 104, 106, 108, 109, 110, 111
intracellular calcium, 4, 40
intramuscular injection, 91
intraocular, 54
intraocular pressure, 54
intravenously, 41
ion channels, 40
ionization, 31
IR spectra, 154
iron, 153, 155, 156, 157, 166
irritability, 52, 56, 63, 66, 69
isolation, 122
isotherms, xi, 140, 189
Israel, 94, 104, 107

K

KBr, 154, 160
kidney(s), 49, 115, 167
kidney stones, 167
kinase activity, 121, 131, 133
kinetics, 129, 153, 162, 174

L

labeling, 102
laboratory studies, 57, 99
lactate level, 63
latency, 96, 97
LDL, 50, 81
lead, 8, 96, 98, 101, 121, 122, 152, 153, 154, 175
learning, 22, 48
legislation, 102
lesions, 9, 17
lever-press training, 22, 23
light, viii, 3, 15, 19, 21, 22, 23, 24, 48, 57, 67, 80, 85, 98, 104
lignin, 158
linear model, 68
lipid metabolism, 54
lipolysis, 62
liquid phase, 143, 146, 166, 189
liquids, 199
liver, viii, 35, 38, 53, 56, 74, 75, 76, 86, 115, 121, 129, 136
liver cirrhosis, 74, 86
liver disease, viii, 35, 56, 76
localization, 133, 135
locomotor, 21, 28, 31, 32, 33, 34, 100, 105, 111
LSD, 96
lumbar puncture, 74
lung function, 49

J

Japan, 113
jaundice, 53

M

macromolecules, 143
macronutrients, 40

Index

magnesium, 153
magnetic resonance, 8
magnetic resonance imaging, 8
magnitude, 73
major depression, 64
majority, 20, 39, 99, 167, 171, 172
mammalian cells, 134
man, 86
management, 57, 129
manganese, 153
mania, 66, 84
manic, 66, 84
manufacturing, 140, 194, 195
marketing, 56, 90, 102
masking, 101
mass, 31, 143, 148, 152, 166, 192
mass spectrometry, 31
mateine, vii, 36
materials, xi, 139, 154, 174, 175, 176, 195
matrix, 160
MB, 11, 12
measurement(s), 3, 144, 145,146, 166, 167,
    175, 177, 178, 179, 181, 182, 183, 184,
    186, 189, 197
meat, 76
media, 143, 175
median, 58
mediation, 30, 133
medical, 37, 67, 69, 98
medicine, 60, 83, 167
melatonin, 14
mellitus, 115
melting, 182
memory, 6, 7, 8, 9, 11, 13, 14, 15, 48, 60,
    85, 99, 105
menstrual cycles, 51
mental disorder, 63, 64, 67, 68, 69
mercury, 145
meta-analysis, 16, 52, 75, 85, 86, 128
Metabolic, 75, 76, 85, 128, 133
metabolic acidosis, 57
metabolic changes, x, 114
metabolic disorder(s), 130, 133
metabolic disturbances, 57, 136
metabolic pathways, 62

metabolic syndrome, 51
metabolism, ix, 2, 17, 38, 39, 40, 56, 75, 76,
    77, 91, 103, 113, 115, 125, 126, 128,
    129, 130, 132, 133, 135, 138
metabolites, 38, 40
metabolized, viii, 35, 56, 74
metastasis, 55
meter, 155, 176
methanol, 201
methyl group, 47
methylation, 43
methylxanthine, viii, 35, 39, 132
Mexico, 102
Mg^{2+}, 167
Miami, 1
mice, 6, 13, 14, 33, 91, 94, 95, 96, 97, 103,
    104, 105, 107, 108, 109, 122, 129, 133,
    136
microcrystalline, 155, 158, 159, 176
microcrystalline cellulose, 155, 158, 159,
    176
microphotographs, 151
microscope, 144, 154
microscopy, 194
microsomes, 38
migraine headache, 73
military, 2
mineralization, 154
miosis, 54
mitochondria, 7, 14
mixing, xi, 95, 98, 102, 108, 140, 146, 175,
    177, 179, 189
models, 14, 70, 77, 93, 101, 110, 116, 175
moisture, 144
moisture content, 144
molar volume, 189
mold, 152, 154
mole, 177, 179, 186
molecular dynamics, 175
molecular structure, 175
molecular weight, 179
molecules, 38, 118, 160, 197
mood change, 65, 66
mood disorder, 9
morbidity, 54

morphine, 74, 86, 91, 103, 107, 110
morphology, 162, 194, 197
mortality, 52, 54, 58, 59, 75
mortality risk, 59
Moscow, 198, 201
motivation, viii, 19, 21, 23, 26, 27, 28, 95
motor activity, 66, 107
motor task, 59
MR, 11, 12, 82
MRI, 15
multivariate analysis, 58
muscle contraction, 4, 115, 119, 127, 133, 134, 135
muscle performance, 18
muscles, x, 5, 62, 114, 119, 120, 122, 123, 124, 126
musculoskeletal, 50
musculoskeletal system, 50
mutation, 55, 137
myocardial infarction, 80
myocardium, 5, 12
myoclonus, 50
myocyte, 4
myopathy, 57

N

NaCl, 198
NAD, 138
National Health and Nutrition Examination Survey, 82
National Institute of Mental Health, 102
National Institutes of Health, 22, 30
nausea, 47, 50, 57, 69
necrosis, 131
negative consequences, 98, 99, 104
negative effects, 102
nephropathy, 54
nerve, 80
nervous system, 47, 48, 56, 58, 62, 85, 94, 104
nervousness, 53, 56, 64, 66, 67
neurologic performance, ix, 36
neurons, 14
neuropharmacology, 31

neuroscience, 105
neurotoxicity, 13
neurotransmission, 30
neurotransmitter(s), 6, 40, 64, 94
nickel, 156, 157
nicotinamide, 31
nicotine, viii, 19, 20, 21, 28, 29, 32, 33, 34, 77, 91, 109, 110, 111
nodes, 131
non-institutionalized, 3
nonsmokers, 91
non-smokers, 70
norepinephrine, 47, 71
Norway, 102
NSAIDs, 77
nucleus, 31, 32, 47
nutrients, 153
nutrition, 11, 12, 17, 77

O

obesity, 76, 129, 131, 132
ofloxacin, 77
OH, 158
oil, 200
olanzapine, 76
old age, 6, 8, 17
omeprazole, 76
operant conditioning, 22
opiates, 91
organ, ix, 113
organic compounds, 201
organic solvents, 141, 194
organism, 40, 41, 71, 153, 167
organs, 47, 115
osteoporosis, 54, 81
overweight, 81
ovulation, 51
oxalate, 167
oxidation, 122, 127, 134
oxidative stress, 14, 135
oxygen, 71

Index   213

P

pain, vii, 1, 5, 12, 13, 57, 61, 80
pain perception, 5, 12, 13
palpitations, 48, 57, 64, 66
pancreatic cancer, 55
panic attack, 53, 64, 65
panic disorder, 65
parallel, 179
parents, 131
parkinsonism, 110
paroxetine, 76, 77
participants, 2, 4, 8, 9, 59, 99
patents, 141, 142
pathogenesis, 7
pathology, 14
pathophysiological, 82
pathways, 6, 39, 118, 122, 123, 126, 131
perceived control, 101
perfusion, 15
permeability, 135
permission, 117, 119, 124
petroleum, 141
pH, 62, 63
pharmaceutical, 194, 197, 200
pharmacokinetics, 2, 74, 86
pharmacology, 78, 135
phase diagram, 200
phenolic compounds, 75
Philadelphia, 84
phosphate, 121
phosphorus, 153
phosphorylation, x, 47, 114, 116, 117, 118,
    119, 120, 121, 122, 123, 124, 126, 130,
    131, 132, 135, 137
physical activity, 2, 17
physical chemistry, 198, 199
physical performance, vii, 1, 2, 3, 4, 9, 61
physical properties, 159, 181
Physiological, 12
physiological arousal, 15
PI3K, 116, 118, 121
pilot study, 108
placebo, 2, 3, 4, 5, 8, 10, 11, 48, 60, 63, 70,
    71, 85, 86

plants, 37, 41, 42, 43, 63, 153
plasma membrane, 116
plasma proteins, 38
platform, 2, 145
playing, ix, 113
pleasure, 5, 12
plexus, 7
PM, 22, 34, 82, 86, 97, 177, 182
poison, 167
polar, 39
polycyclic aromatic hydrocarbon, 76
polymer(s), 143, 155, 175
polymer materials, 143
polyphenols, 140, 143
population, 3, 4, 8, 17, 39, 63, 67, 70, 81,
    84, 90
Portugal, 8, 16
positive correlation, 92
positive mood, 64, 65
potassium, 4, 12, 40, 153, 167
potential benefits, 48, 64
preeclampsia, 52
prefrontal cortex, 31
pregnancy, viii, 35, 50, 52, 76
prematurity, ix, 35, 71, 80, 85
preparation, 36, 41, 154, 160
preservation, 9
pressure gauge, 145
preterm infants, 49, 85
prevention, 71, 80, 115, 117, 126
priming, 29
principles, 51
probability, 77, 98
processing biases, 15
prochlorperazine, ix, 36
procurement, 26
producers, 37
profit, 141
proliferation, 92
proteins, 7, 116, 130
psychiatric disorders, 64, 65
psychiatric patients, 70, 83
psychopathology, 53
psychosis, 53, 54, 57, 66, 84
psychosocial stress, 14

214 Index

psychostimulants, 60, 68, 83
psychotic symptoms, 53, 64, 65, 66
public health, 98, 102, 104, 107
pulmonary edema, 57
pumps, 145
pure water, 144
purification, 166
purity, 144, 166, 176, 181
pyridoxine, 31

Q

quartile, 8
quercetin, 15
questioning, 178
questionnaire, 7, 9

R

Rab, 116
racing, 11, 57, 66
raw materials, xi, 139, 151, 152, 155, 162, 166, 167, 173
RE, 32
reaction time, 3, 7, 13, 15, 48, 99, 100, 107
reactions, 52, 56
reactive oxygen, 7
reactivity, 143
reading, 8
reasoning, 7, 48, 60
recall, 99
receptors, 6, 7, 13, 30, 31, 32, 33, 39, 40, 48, 49, 50, 60, 63, 64, 77, 79, 94, 103, 104, 106, 108
recognition, 6, 13, 14
recommendations, 72
recovery, 56, 66, 146, 200
recreational, 101
recrystallization, 197
recycling, 142
redistribution, 56
regulatory agencies, 56
rehydration, 143

reinforcement, viii, 19, 22, 23, 25, 31, 33, 64, 68, 94
reintroduction, 96
relaxation, 50, 175
relevance, 29, 110
reliability, 175, 177
relief, 68, 73
researchers, 51, 55, 59, 125
residues, 116
resistance, 5, 12, 117, 118
resolution, 144, 154
respiration, 49
respiratory disorders, 49
respiratory failure, 67
response, x, 3, 18, 22, 23, 24, 25, 28, 29, 31, 34, 58, 60, 72, 75, 86, 96, 104, 114, 118, 121, 122, 126, 129
restrictions, 102
restructuring, 160
reticulum, 5, 62, 125
retinopathy, 71
rewards, 20, 21, 26, 29
rhabdomyolysis, 50, 57, 81
rheumatoid arthritis, 167
rhythm, 48, 57
riboflavin, 31
righting, 109
rings, 158
risk(s), 8, 9, 16, 17, 49, 50, 51, 52, 53, 54, 55, 56, 58, 59, 65, 67, 73, 74, 75, 76, 79, 80, 81, 82, 83, 85, 86, 87, 92, 93, 98, 99, 101, 103, 108, 109, 115, 116, 128
risk assessment, 99
rodents, ix, 28, 34, 60, 89, 93, 95, 100, 109, 132
rotations, 159, 160
rules, 102
Russia, 139, 140

S

safety, 74, 153
saliva, 39, 74, 86
salts, 141, 167, 171, 172, 173
saturation, 39, 146, 178, 183

Index

savings, 144
schizophrenia, 64, 66, 84
school, 54, 201
school performance, 54
science, 12
secretion, 47, 50, 54
sedative, 77, 94, 99
sedatives, 70, 83
seed, 41
seizure, ix, 35
selenium, 153
semen, 39
semiconductor, 154
sensing, 132
sensitivity, 40, 49, 71, 108, 127
sensitization, 105
serine, 117, 118, 131, 132
serotonin, 48, 60, 77
serotonin syndrome, 77
serum, 5, 8, 10, 16, 38, 40, 58
sex, ix, 35, 56, 94, 98
showing, 28, 30, 53, 99, 119
side effects, vii, ix, 36, 74
signal transduction, 125, 131
signaling pathway, x, 114, 115, 126, 134
signalling, 131, 135
signs, 67, 85, 91, 99, 101, 103, 107
silica, 146
skeletal muscle, ix, x, 5, 12, 55, 62, 71, 114,
    115, 116, 117, 118, 119, 120, 121, 122,
    123, 124, 125, 126, 128, 130, 131, 132,
    133, 134, 135, 136, 137, 138
sleep deprivation, 7, 15, 47, 63, 64, 71, 85
sleep disorders, 65
sleep disturbance, 52, 66
sleep latency, 66, 95, 105
small intestine, 37
smoking, 52, 76, 109
smooth muscle, 50
soccer, 18
sociability, 69
social acceptance, 54
social anxiety, 65
society, 11, 115
socioeconomic status, 8, 16

sodium, 153, 167
soft drinks, vii, 36, 37, 45, 49, 53, 63
software, 22
soleus, 122, 132, 135
solid phase, 152, 153, 166
solubility, xi, 140, 144, 145, 146, 147, 148,
    155, 189, 198, 200
solution, 63, 96, 141, 146, 152, 153, 189,
    192, 193, 194, 197
solvents, 141, 143, 196
somnolence, 73
South America, vii, 36, 42
SP, 84
Spain, 78, 89, 96, 102
specialists, 194
species, vii, 7, 36, 41
specific heat, 184
speech, 67
spinal anesthesia, 74
spinal puncture headache, ix, 35
spine, 14
spontaneous abortion, 51
Sprague-Dawley rats, viii, 19, 21
SS, 34
St. Petersburg, 197
stability, 175
stabilization, 146
state(s), 4, 17, 18, 37, 60, 64, 72, 90, 117,
    144, 154, 175, 178, 199, 200
steel, 145
stimulant, 28, 30, 32, 33, 34, 47, 49, 60, 62,
    63, 64, 71, 72, 80, 99, 100, 103, 105, 140
stimulation, x, 5, 32, 39, 49, 55, 62, 99, 108,
    114, 122, 126, 134, 137
stimulus, viii, 5, 19, 21, 23, 26, 28, 29, 32,
    33
stock, 148
stomach, 37
stress, 6, 23, 33, 82, 95, 104, 131, 133
stretching, 158, 159, 160
striatum, 15
stroke, 75, 101, 108
structural changes, 151, 153, 162, 169, 172
structure, xi, 38, 133, 140, 143, 152, 155,
    159, 166, 175, 191, 196, 197, 199

216 Index

substance use, 70
substitution, 29, 99
substrate, ix, x, 89, 114, 116, 123, 125, 130, 131, 132, 135
substrates, 122, 131
sucrose, 28, 29, 34
sulfate, 167
sulfur, 141, 153
sulfur dioxide, 141
sulfuric acid, 167
Sun, 129, 132
supplementation, 12
suppression, 101, 118
supraventricular tachycardia, 53
survival, 71
susceptibility, 56, 68
Sweden, 55
swelling, 144, 152, 167, 172, 175, 192, 194
sympathetic nervous system, 62
symptoms, 55, 57, 59, 64, 65, 66, 67, 68, 69, 70, 72, 73, 76, 85, 95, 101
synapse, 7
synaptic plasticity, 15
syndrome, 51, 65, 66, 68, 69, 70, 74, 84, 136
synergistic effect, 11
synthesis, 4, 43, 48, 94, 115, 122, 127, 130
systolic blood pressure, 52

T

tachycardia, 47, 53, 55, 57, 64, 66, 67
tachypnea, 57
Taiwan, 105
target, 60, 126, 133, 143, 148, 167, 169, 174, 176, 194
team sports, 2
technical assistance, 30
technology, 142, 194, 195, 199
temperature, xi, 21, 140, 142, 146, 148, 150, 151, 155, 169, 171, 175, 178, 179, 181, 182, 183, 184, 187, 188, 189, 190, 191, 193, 200
tension, 9, 69, 73, 107
tension headache, 73

test procedure, 30
test scores, 8
testing, 9, 95
thalamus, 64
theine, vii, 36, 140
theophylline, viii, 31, 35, 38, 47, 76, 77, 81, 101, 107, 132, 200
therapeutic effects, 66, 101
therapy, ix, 36, 71, 74, 80
thermal analysis, 200
thermal expansion, 177
thermal stability, 200
thermodynamic equilibrium, 146
thermodynamic properties, 199
thermodynamic systems, xi, 140
thoughts, 66
tin, 56
tinnitus, 67
tissue, 119, 124
tobacco, 51, 70, 87, 110, 143, 196
tonic, 67
total cholesterol, 50
total energy, 40
toxic effect, 56
toxicity, ix, 5, 36, 56, 57, 77, 82
toxicology, 135
training, 22, 61, 62, 72, 129, 138, 194
transcription, 137
transesterification, 201
transformations, 160
translocation, 116, 121, 130, 133
transmission, ix, 66, 90
transport, ix, x, 7, 114, 115, 116, 117, 118, 119, 120, 121, 122, 123, 124, 125, 126, 130, 133, 134, 135, 136, 192
treatment, 6, 15, 20, 37, 48, 49, 53, 57, 66, 71, 73, 84, 85, 97, 101, 106, 115, 123, 136, 141, 143, 146, 152, 154, 156, 157, 158, 159, 161, 171, 173, 174, 175, 194, 196, 199
tremor, 50, 53, 64, 66, 110
trial, vii, 1, 2, 4, 5, 7, 10, 11, 12, 71, 73, 86
triggers, 116
triglycerides, 50
tumor, 55, 134

Index

217

tumor cells, 55
type 2 diabetes, 59, 75, 87, 128, 129, 130
tyrosine, x, 6, 114, 116, 117, 118, 120, 121, 133

U

UK, 102
United States, 20, 32, 80, 82, 90
urine, 2, 39, 49, 53, 62
USA, 199
UV, 144

V

vacuum, 145
validation, 85
valve, 178
vapor, 189
variables, 101
variations, 39, 167, 171, 184
varieties, 42, 43
vasoconstriction, 48, 51
vasodilation, 49
vegetable oil, 201
vegetables, 76, 143
vein, 120, 124
velocity, 8, 10
venlafaxine, 77
ventricular arrhythmias, 53, 80
vessels, 141
vibration, 158, 160
viscosity, 141
vision, 102
visual attention, 11, 31
visual processing, 10
vitamin C, 153
vitamins, 153
VLA, 177, 182

vomiting, 47, 57, 58, 69
vulnerability, 70

W

walking, 2, 100
Washington, 67, 69, 83, 85, 103
water, xi, 22, 41, 42, 96, 97, 140, 141, 142, 148, 149, 151, 152, 155, 158, 166, 176, 179, 196, 197, 198, 200
water purification, 155
weakness, 57
weight gain, 51
weight loss, 57, 115, 129
well-being, 63, 110
western blot, 119, 124
white matter, 9, 17
withdrawal, vii, ix, 1, 3, 15, 32, 36, 54, 55, 59, 62, 64, 65, 68, 69, 70, 74, 85, 91, 95, 96, 97, 103, 104, 107, 110
withdrawal symptoms, 59, 68, 69, 70
workers, 72, 80
working conditions, 167
working memory, 8, 15
working population, 105
worldwide, vii, 2, 36, 115

Y

yield, xi, 139
young adults, 92
young people, 90, 93, 98, 101

Z

zinc, 153, 154, 156, 157